Praise for
Climbing Higher

"[Montel Williams] is revealing it all in [*Climbing Higher*]. It's an absolutely riveting read not only for his fans, but for anyone who's ever suffered from serious illness."   —*New York Post*

"Here [Montel Williams] displays his resolve not to be beaten down but to lead a vital and productive life."   —*Library Journal*

"Montel Williams is determined to help people with multiple sclerosis—he is equally determined not to let his own MS interfere with his enjoyment of life."   —*The Dallas Morning News*

Montel
Williams
WITH LAWRENCE GROBEL

Climbing
Higher

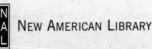

NEW AMERICAN LIBRARY

New American Library
Published by New American Library, a division of
Penguin Group (USA) Inc., 375 Hudson Street,
New York, New York 10014, USA
Penguin Group (Canada), 10 Alcorn Avenue,Toronto,
Ontario, M4V 3B2, Canada (a division of Pearson Penguin Canada Inc.)
Penguin Books Ltd., 80 Strand, London WC2R 0RL, England
Penguin Ireland, 25 St. Stephen's Green, Dublin 2,
Ireland (a division of Penguin Books Ltd.)
Penguin Group (Australia), 250 Camberwell Road, Camberwell, Victoria 3124,
Australia (a division of Pearson Australia Group Pty. Ltd.)
Penguin Books India Pvt. Ltd., 11 Community Centre, Panchsheel Park,
New Delhi - 110 017, India
Penguin Group (NZ), cnr Airborne and Rosedale Roads, Albany,
Auckland 1310, New Zealand (a division of Pearson New Zealand Ltd.)
Penguin Books (South Africa) (Pty.) Ltd., 24 Sturdee Avenue,
Rosebank, Johannesburg 2196, South Africa

Penguin Books Ltd., Registered Offices:
80 Strand, London WC2R 0RL, England

Published by New American Library,
a division of Penguin Group (USA) Inc. Previously published in a
New American Library hardcover edition.

First New American Library Trade Paperback Printing, January 2005
1 3 5 7 9 10 8 6 4 2

NEW AMERICAN LIBRARY and logo are trademarks of Penguin Group (USA) Inc.

New American Library Trade Paperback ISBN: 0-451-21398-X

THE LIBRARY OF CONGRESS HAS CATALOGUED THE HARDCOVER EDITION AS FOLLOWS:

Williams, Montel.
    Climbing higher/Montel Williams with Lawrence Grobel.
       p.   cm.
    ISBN 0-451-21159-6
    1. Williams, Montel.   2. Television personalities—United States—Biography.   I.
Grobel, Lawrence.   II. Title.
PN1992.4.W553A3 2004
791.4502'8'092—dc22   2003021905

Set in Sabon
Designed by Lenny Telesca

Printed in the United States of America

PUBLISHER'S NOTE
Every effort has been made to ensure that the information contained in this book is complete and accurate. However, neither the publisher nor the author is engaged in rendering
professional advice or services to the individual reader. The ideas, procedures, and sugges-
tions contained in this book are not intended as a substitute for consulting with your
physician. All matters regarding your health require medical supervision. Neither the
author nor the publisher shall be liable or responsible for any loss or damage allegedly arising from any information or suggestion in this book. The opinions expressed in this book
represent the personal views of the author and not of the publisher.

For Wyntergrace, Montel, Maressa, and Ashley,
for really, truly loving me, without question.
You were my reason to get up off that street—and
to keep from ever going there again.

Contents

Acknowledgments

It's hard to climb a mountain on your own. There are people you need along the way, and I've been extremely fortunate to have a lot of good people supporting me. I want to thank them for being there when I've needed them. Without them, I wouldn't be scaling heights at all.

So thank you to Melanie McLaughlin—my sister, my daughter, my confidante, my rock. Jennifer Roe-Reyes, who babysits me like no other personal assistant could. Dawn McNiff, the best nanny any adult could ever have and a damn good friend. Nina Shaw, the best attorney in the business—thanks for thirteen great years and here's to another thirteen. Angela Lee, for your continued support, both professionally and personally. Cheryl McCourtie and Nancy Goldman, who stepped in and helped turn a dream into a foundation. Guy, Joe and Rupert—you know my dogs run deep. Dr. S. Allen Counter, who I will always feel indebted to for helping me spend more time with my family. Tracy Bernstein, my editor, for her precision and attention to detail. Maya Grobel, without whose tireless work, no deadline would have been met. Jennifer Johnson-Spence, a dedicated librarian who was so willing and able to provide research for a complex issue.

And to Tara Westwood, for setting the standard for what I seek in love. I'm forever indebted to you for helping me understand how important it is for me to see the truth.

Special thanks to Larry Grobel, without whom there would be no book. You've taken me on a journey that I hadn't anticipated going on. From the first day we sat down to talk, I knew I was blessed to have gotten you to do this. You've given me the chance to give some meaning to what has happened to me since being diagnosed. I would recommend you as a therapist to just about anybody. It's an understatement to say this book has been cathartic and healing.

Prologue

The title of my first book, *Mountain, Get Out of My Way*, was my battle cry. It's a biblical reference—Matthew 17:20: "If ye have faith as a grain of mustard seed, ye shall say unto this mountain, 'Remove hence to yonder place;' and it shall remove; and nothing shall be impossible unto you."

Every speech I made I began with that phrase—Mountain, get out of my way!—in a loud, booming voice. It said that no matter how great an obstacle you think is facing you—if you're the product of a broken family, if a parent or friend has died, if you're in serious trouble—no matter what that obstacle or impediment may be in your life, all you really need is true faith in yourself and an understanding of who you are, and you can overcome it.

When I speak around the country to kids, one of the things I most want them to hear is that if you have faith in yourself, you don't have to live up to *or down to* anyone else's expectations. Faith in yourself allows you to truly own the definition of who you are. That's my center, my rock. No one is going to tell me what I'm going to be like—as a father, as a talk show host, as an actor, or as a person with MS. I know what I want to be and I will do my best to live up to my definition. *Mountain, Get Out of My Way* expresses that.

In that first book I talked a lot about trying my best to move
obstacles out of my way. I told some stories, but my intention was to
be motivational, not self-revealing. I wasn't even 20 percent as open
as I am in this one. That first book made the bestseller list, so I guess
people liked it, but I didn't give up a lot of me. With this one, while
I hope it may help others with MS or any other chronic or deadly
disease, I've finally realized something: I could go on barreling
ahead, eyes front, shoulders hunched, trying to mow down obstacles, and I'd certainly get *somewhere*, but am I sure it's where I truly
want to go? I can push, knock, kick and scream away all the obstacles I want, but that's not going to take me any higher.

Before, I wanted to move mountains. Now I'd like to stand at the
top of a mountain and look around. That's what this is about: to
stop, take a look, get some perspective. I may have pushed a lot of
mountains away, but I didn't really conquer them. For that, I don't
just have to get around them, but over them. It's time to climb a little higher, take a clear look around and see where I am.

1

"You Have MS."

I'm in the intensive care unit of Beth Israel North waiting to go into surgery, where I have a 50 percent chance of dying. The blood vessel leading to my sinuses is ten times the size it should be and blood has been pouring out of my nose for nearly a month. There are tubes going in and out of me, connected to a heart monitor. The cauterization inside my nose suddenly bursts and blood starts shooting like a jet stream across the bed. I look at the heart monitor and see the numbers go from 65 to 58, to 50, 40, 29. My blood pressure is 80/10. The monitor starts making noises and just before it flatlines I shout for the doctor. I don't want to die, but the machine shows 0 as I pass out. I'm dead.

But somehow I'm aware of what's going on around me and I'm freaked out. There are four doctors trying to revive me. And one stranger, a strange sort of apparition cloaked in a shroud. Is it an angel? Am I going to be escorted to the white light? The figure approaches me and softly says, "Montel, Montel, you need to calm the fuck down."

The doctors aren't aware of this stranger. I don't know who he is—I'm not even sure it's a he—but he's not like any angel I ever imagined. Whoever it is, it makes me laugh.

"What are you talking about?" I say. I'm laughing because here *is my big deathbed scene and I get an angel with a filthy mouth. I'm dying and he's telling me to stay calm?*

"You heard me," he says again. "If I don't tell it to you this way you are not going to listen. So calm the fuck down. It's not your time. You've still got too many things to accomplish." One of the doctors, Dr. Swarup, grabs my chest with his fingers and twists my skin hard enough to leave a bruise. "Montel!" he shouts. "Wake up! Wake up!"

Another doctor starts yelling as well. "Who are you talking to? You've got to calm down!"

"That's what he just said," I murmur and point to the apparition. When I finally calm down, I look up and it's gone. My four doctors bring me back.

The next morning the anesthesiologist comes to prepare me for surgery. I say to her, "Make sure I wake up from this." I want to live. I'm not sure if what happened the day before is something that I imagined to ease my concern about dying or if it was truly a visitation, but I feel a sense of calm that I haven't felt for a very long time.

It isn't going to last.

Ten months later, in February of 1999, I flew to Salt Lake City, Utah, to appear in an episode of the TV show *Touched by an Angel*. On the plane, I got up to use the bathroom, and when I returned I stumbled and fell into the seat next to Grace, my wife. Our relationship was not at a high point and now what the hell was this? A searing pain had swept through my legs from the knees to the feet as if they had been scalded by a blowtorch. It wasn't a momentary fire but a continuous one. My feet felt like someone had taken a sharp, pointed branding iron and stuck it not just between my toes but through them. The pain was so excruciating I didn't think I would be able to walk, let alone act. But I also knew that I had made a commitment to do the show and I felt obligated to honor that commitment.

I work out with a trainer every morning, and a day earlier I had trained with somebody new doing a different type of leg workout. I thought that I must have done something horribly wrong in my workout. Every hour for the next two days, my legs and feet hurt more. We were staying with a very close friend of mine, Dr. Andy Hines, who is a plastic surgeon. I told him about the pain and that I thought I might have really screwed up my back. By then my feet had gone numb, as had a small spot on my side from my hip to the bottom of my rib cage. I also felt pain in my stomach that was taking my breath away. Andy told Grace he suspected I had a neurological disorder but he didn't say anything to me because he knew I had to work the next day.

I didn't want to tell anybody that I was hurting the first day on the set because then they'd have to cancel the shoot, and that would probably be the last guest-starring appearance I'd ever get. So I took six Tylenol, sucked it up and went to work. When anyone asked what was wrong, I said I pinched a nerve in my back from working out and it would be no problem.

It should have been a fun shoot. It was a beautiful day. The air was clear, the sun was shining. My love interest was Cynthia Nixon, who had just signed a deal for *Sex and the City*. I was playing a juicy role, a cult leader who was destined to go straight to hell. We had two tough scenes that day. One was the opening, in which I was recruiting people to come with me to my compound. I had to walk up and down the aisles in front of twenty or thirty people giving a long speech. If you ever see this episode, don't be fooled; what may appear to be intense Acting with a capital A is actually physical pain. Every step I took was so painful I had to clasp my hands in front of me and squeeze as hard as I could to deflect how much my feet hurt.

I got back to Andy's around five p.m. and collapsed. I had the next day off, which was a relief because I woke up in even worse pain. "I really want you to go see a friend of mine," Andy said. "He's a neurologist and he may be able to explain some of this." Then he casually asked if anyone had ever mentioned multiple sclerosis to me.

"Yeah," I said, "but I know it's not that. Twenty years ago I had a doctor in the marines suggest I should be tested for MS. Turned out it disappeared. Six years ago, same thing: this doctor in Las Vegas put me through an MRI [magnetic resonance imager], thought it was MS, sent me to an eye clinic in Philadelphia. The top doctor there looked at the MRI and said those people were crazy: it wasn't MS—it was an inner-ear infection I had caught from swimming in the bay. Once these doctors see the kind of shape I'm in and understand the kind of power weight lifting I do, they know I'm no victim of disease. I just get these damn pains and need something to stop them."

I looked at Andy and saw he wasn't buying it. And that kind of took me aback, because I am where I am today because of my self-assurance, the power of my conviction; it's the power of who I am. If Albert Einstein were alive today and came on my show, I probably could argue him out of being so sure that e equals mc squared.

But there was no talking my way out of the pain I was feeling, so Andy's sister-in-law Wendy drove me to the neurologist in Salt Lake City. She had to drive because I was hurting so bad I could not put my foot on the gas pedal.

The doctor's office was in one of those executive centers that look like a strip mall. I was expecting him to give me some pain medication and send me on my way. I wasn't expecting him to turn my life upside down.

He said that from what Andy had told him and seeing me walk, he knew exactly what was wrong, but he didn't say what it was and I didn't ask. He did a quick eye exam, holding up fingers for me to count; told me to bend over; and had me remove my pants so he could conduct some needle tests to check my legs.

I told him I had been on some medication for the past few months because I had been urinating a lot. I also said that I was having trouble releasing my bowels—I would try to go six times in a row but nothing happened. He just nodded. These were classic symptoms of the disease I didn't yet know I had.

He began sticking needles into my feet.

"What do you feel?"

"Nothing."

He poked me in the legs, drawing blood. "Do you feel this?"

"No."

He poked some more. I didn't feel anything.

For the first time I began to face how seriously numb I had gone in various places on my body. Two years before this I had burned myself on the space heater in my office, a second-degree burn, and I didn't even know it. I'd had a car back over my foot and didn't realize it until a half hour later when my foot started hurting.

The doctor then checked my cremasteric reflex, which is supposed to make the genitals move when the thigh is touched in a certain spot. Mine didn't.

"I can tell you without doing any further tests that you have MS," he said. Just like that. Very matter-of-fact.

What the hell was he talking about, MS? Even though I'd heard those two letters before, I barely knew what MS was. I thought it was the disease Jerry Lewis was always raising money to defeat. Kids in wheelchairs. I was an adult. I couldn't have that. I didn't know anything about MS. I thought it was muscular dystrophy.

He asked if I knew any other neurologists I trusted. Now I was back on more solid ground. "Sure, I have a doctor at Harvard, Dr. Allen Counter, who could help set up appointments with a neurologist there." He had invited me up to Harvard to speak on African-Americans and minorities in the media two months earlier, and had impressed me as one of the true treasures of this country. He was a neurophysiologist at Harvard Medical School who had been the director of the Harvard Foundation for more than two decades. I was dropping Dr. Counter's name as if to let this doctor know I knew real doctors who could counter his cocksure diagnosis.

"Then you ought to go to Harvard," he said, "because you have MS—there's no question."

I gave him a look of infinite hatred . . . and broke down. Tears have always come easily for me, but this time I was crying at the thought of my own funeral. My kids were going to be robbed of their dad. My hopes of fulfilling the old high school yearbook prediction of one day residing at 1600 Pennsylvania Avenue were instantly crushed. This black man wasn't going to be the first African-American president. He was just going to be one dead talk show host.

My tears clearly made the doctor uncomfortable. "Don't cry," he said. "There's nothing you can do about it."

Thanks a lot, I thought, and I cried even more. I've had doctors look me in the face and just because I had convinced them that they should look somewhere else they changed their minds about their diagnosis. But I suspected this time the doctor might be right that I had a disease. And a disease meant that I wasn't going to ever be the same.

When I finally regained some semblance of composure I asked him, "Where do we go from here?"

"Truthfully?" he said. "You should not exercise because it puts an unnecessary strain on your body. It's not the best idea for you."

"But I'm a weight lifter," I said. "I work out every day."

"Your exercise routines will have to change," he said. "First, you must wait until this bout has gone. Then, see your doctor at Harvard."

I tried to protest that his diagnosis might be wrong. Doctors today often second-guess themselves because they don't want to get sued. And with a disease like MS, where the symptoms can come and go, being in remission could potentially validate that I was misdiagnosed. But he wouldn't back down, saying, again, in that painfully matter-of-fact way: "Go ahead and see your Harvard doctor, and he will confirm what I've just told you. You have MS. You will have to learn how to live with it."

I didn't like the cocky manner this doctor had. I didn't like the blunt way he diagnosed me. But most of all I didn't like him because he was the messenger, and what he was telling me was that my life was about to change. He was suggesting I go from being a strong healthy man to a weak, ill patient. He was telling me, without saying it, that I had better prepare myself to become a cripple. That my days of bodybuilding would become months and years of body breakdown. He poked and stabbed my numb lower body and showed me that what was in store for me was either excruciating pain or no feeling whatsoever. He was pronouncing my death sentence. I was forty-three years old and he was telling me that I was going to die.

I didn't want him to tell anybody. I made sure we were clear about doctor-patient privilege before I went out to the car, where Wendy was waiting. Immediately I called Dr. Counter on my cell phone and left a message saying I needed some help. Wendy asked if I was okay.

"Yeah, yeah—everything's okay."

When we got back to Andy's house I pulled Andy and his wife, Kim, aside and said, "You can't say anything to anybody; our entire friendship really hinges on this. If this gets out I'll know it's you." We all got emotional. They hugged me and told me over and over, "It's not the end of the world," while I let loose all my fears.

"What am I going to do? I don't want my kids to know. I don't want anyone to know. I'll lose my job. I'll never get asked to act again. I'm going to die."

We started pulling out books, reading anything in the house we could find about MS. I learned that there were four different stages: benign, regressive, relapsing-remitting, and progressive. I assumed I must be progressive, the worst category, because I wasn't bad the week before, and the pain in my legs was just getting worse.

At the same time, as much as I was thinking the worst, I was trying my best to act normal—I still had to finish the episode of *Touched by an Angel*. I finally got Dr. Counter on the phone and he suggested that we immediately set up an appointment with two of Harvard's top MS doctors, Dr. Howard Weiner and Dr. Michael Olek, and in the interim, get some Vicodin pain pills. I took five in an hour and they barely helped, other than putting my brain in a whole other place.

All day Wednesday I was cloudy and had a little bit of a problem remembering my lines, but I tried my best to hide my pain and numbness. I kept up the charade that I had a back problem and everyone accepted it. I was feeling so bad and so weak that I decided not to listen to the doctor and went to the gym before shooting the last two days. I used every ounce of strength to do it, but I worked out. When we shot the climactic scene in which the angel and I do battle and I get set on fire, the script called for me to cry. It was the easiest acting I've ever had to do. I just let go on the set; I cried for a day and a half. Everyone was saying what a great actor I was and I let them—thanks, yes, I appreciate that—but those tears weren't fake—I was grieving for my life.

As soon as the episode wrapped Grace and I flew to Boston, where Dr. Counter set me up with Dr. Michael Olek. I kept saying to

Grace about the Salt Lake City doctor, "Well, maybe this guy's wrong."

Dr. Olek was about five feet eight inches and looked like he was thirteen years old. But he had an impressive number of diplomas hanging on the wall behind his desk. He gave me a thorough clinical examination as I ranted and raved about how much of a jerk the other doctor was and generally made it clear he better not treat me that way. He checked my hands, eyes, ears, face, tongue and throat. He listened to my speech. He checked each leg from heel to shin. He used a pin, and a tuning fork. He checked my motor skills. Then he put me through the MRI, a multimillion-dollar scanner that uses magnetic fields up to 30,000 times stronger than the earth's radio-wave pulses to produce pictures of the central nervous system—far more specific than those produced by CAT scanners or X-rays. These sequential pictures of the brain and spinal cord show wafer-thin slices of the tissue, making it possible to detect extremely small lesions and areas of demyelination, or damaged nerve fibers. He said it would answer definitively whether I had MS.

He called me in and showed me my images. There were multiple scars on my brain.

In a very calming way he said, "Unfortunately, I have confirmed your diagnosis, so let's talk about this."

He explained that multiple sclerosis means multiple scars and pointed out each one on my MRI. "You don't have a lot. Some people come in here for the first time and their brain is already riddled. You have a combination of multiple sclerosis and lateral sclerosis, which means you also have a couple of scars or plaques on your spinal cord as well as on your brain." He sat back in his chair and waited for me to say something, but I had nothing to say. I knew I couldn't run from the answer this time. I appreciated that he was to the point without being insensitive. Finally I asked, "What are we going to do about it?"

"There's nothing we can do to cure you," he said, "but there are three medications out there—they're called the ABC drugs— Avonex, Betaseron and Copaxone." I had read about them. All three were injectable, and all of them had side effects like chest and joint pain, anxiety, muscle stiffness, tissue destruction, fever, chills, depression.

"In a way, you're a lucky man," he said. An odd choice of words, I thought. I wasn't feeling very lucky. "It really all depends on how you look at it. If the severity is rated from one to ten, I'd say you're between a two and three in the number of scars or plaques you have. You definitely have some symptoms, but it doesn't necessarily mean the disease is progressing."

For the next hour he explained everything he knew as a neurologist about this disease. When he started talking about proteins and about the immune system and the fact that the immune system has turned on itself, I made notes so that when I got home I could do more reading about it. "We don't understand it but we think it has something to do with the T2 or T3 thymus lymphocytes, which are immune cells that are near the thyroid," he said. I told him I had a thyroid problem, that I had had a blood test and found that my thyroid level was so low it needed to be augmented with medication. Dr. Olek said that the thymus lymphocytes were a separate issue, but he took note of this because thyroid problems are a potential symptom of MS.

He explained the four categories of MS again and said that about three-quarters of MS patients were in the relapsing-remitting category, in which symptoms appear and then disappear. "Considering you walked in the way you did, the shape you're in, obviously we can't use just your MRI as a diagnostic tool to say how far or how bad your illness is," he said, "because you're doing things that other people with the same level of disease might not be doing. Therefore, it is not affecting you the same way—sometimes different areas of the brain compensate for other areas that are damaged, as if your brain rewired around it."

If my brain was able to rewire, then there was hope. I liked Dr. Olek's manner a whole lot more than that of the Salt Lake City doctor, and I began to appreciate how important it is to feel comfortable with your doctor when you're struggling with the unknown. The Salt Lake City doctor told me I shouldn't exercise; Dr. Olek said the opposite. "You exercised before we diagnosed you, and if I didn't diagnose you, you'd still exercise. You've been through this before, you've had periods of weakness in your back and legs, went to the doctor and just changed your workout routine—so that's what you'll do: change it a bit and then see if you can bring it back. You are in the middle of an episode now and I can put you on a steroid drip. Steroids seem to lessen the inflammation and the pain."

"Hell no," I said. "Not now, not tomorrow, not ever." I didn't want to drip steroids into my body. As a bodybuilder I knew the damage they do to your liver and tendons. I had messed with certain steroids and I knew they could screw up your body. Steroids change your metabolism and your physiology. I don't care what any doctor says; there's a change and for me it's never been positive.

"You're the only person who commands the level of pain you're in," he said. "You told me that it seems to be subsiding, but if it comes back as a ten, or one hundred percent, you shouldn't put yourself through it. We can sometimes contain that with medication."

The doctor pointed me toward Web sites and books that would give me more information and resources. I ended up with a huge stack of paper. After I read through it I was more confused about MS than when I started. You could find five different doctors saying five different things. It seemed everyone out there had a theory, but there were no definitive answers about MS.

I read medical journals, pamphlets, books, articles, trying to find out what this disease was all about. It surprised me how many different symptoms there were; but even more, how many different opinions doctors had. That's what blew me out the door. We were closing in on a new millennium and there was no consensus on anything about the disease.

I had taken two weeks off from my talk show to do the episode of *Touched by an Angel*. So as soon as I returned from seeing Dr. Olek I had to go right back to work. I didn't have any kind of a break to deal with my newly diagnosed disease. I do serious issue-oriented shows and we spend a lot of time talking about child abuse, spousal abuse, stalking, diseases, and all those kinds of things. These topics can be emotionally draining, especially when you're hosting and taping three different shows a day.

If ever I needed a pep talk, this was the time. But even my mountain metaphor couldn't snap me out of it. All the other obstacles in
my life suddenly seemed like hills compared to this. I was facing the
Himalayas, staring down Anapurna, with Everest right behind. How
was I going to push these mountains out of my way?

For six weeks after my diagnosis, when I wasn't on camera I was
crying. At night, I was twitching so much I couldn't stay in bed. It
felt like I was walking across hot coals just to get to the bathroom.
All my thoughts were negative: my job was over, I couldn't perform
in the bedroom, my wife was leaving me. I sat around all day thinking everyone was going to find out; people were going to laugh at
me; or they were going to avoid me because they'd think the disease
was contagious.

The voice in my head was never quiet: "I'm going to be left alone;
my kids are no longer going to want to see me; they'll have to push
me around in a wheelchair." I didn't want them to see me like that. I
didn't want to be a burden on anybody. I buried myself in my work
so I didn't have to be around anybody. I avoided talking to people,
to Grace, my kids. I just tried to avoid human contact. I spiraled
into a cataclysmic depression.

I eventually stopped going to the gym. I couldn't pull weights. My
brain would signal "pull" but my left arm couldn't do it. It was just
a mess. I was an emotional wreck. I wasn't eating; I went from over
200 pounds down to 176 in a little over a month. I was worried
beyond belief.

What was there to live for? My marriage was on the rocks; my
body was either numb or on fire and it was only going to get worse.
Whatever was going on with my immune system was messing with my
brain chemically and making me depressed. I was still swallowing
Percocets and Vicodins trying to lessen the pain I was in. I had no
appetite for food, sex, or conversation. I didn't want to see my friends
or family. I couldn't work out. My staff was in dissension. I was hiding my disease from everyone. I felt alone, hopeless, and sorry for
myself. I just kept talking myself into the vortex that was sucking me
down further every day. On multiple occasions I told Grace she should
leave me. I didn't just have low self-esteem—I had no self-esteem.

But what I did have were guns.

A lot of guns.

Nine guns. All registered. All legal.

Nine choices to blow my brains out and end the misery I was in.

Grace was in Los Angeles trying to get some acting work and my mother-in-law was staying at our house in Greenwich, Connecticut, with Montel and Wyntergrace. Ashley and Maressa were with their mother, my first wife. I decided to spread some towels on the floor of our bedroom closet and clean my guns. At least, I wanted to make it appear as if that was what I was doing when they found me there.

It was just past midnight when I went into the walk-in closet and took down my SP89, which is a big semiautomatic handgun, similar to an Uzi. It looks like a Mac 10 and has a big clip that attaches to it. That gun had so much kick, though, that I was afraid when I pulled the trigger it would slip from my hand and wouldn't make a big enough hole. I'd have to shoot myself twice. But what if the gun fell out of my hand? So I took the gun apart—it breaks down into a lot of different parts—and laid it on the towel next to the cleaning fluids.

I next took three 9mm guns out of their cases: the Glock, the Beretta, and the Sigsaur. I held each of them in my hand, but decided that a 9mm wouldn't make a great hole. I wasn't looking to wound myself. So the only other option was the .38 Special or the .357 Magnum. If I pulled the trigger on the Magnum, a cylinder weapon with hydroshock hollow-point bullets in it, there would be nothing left of me.

I broke down the Glock and laid it alongside the SP89 and looked at the remaining guns on the towels and in their cases. It had to be the .357. No matter where I shot myself with that one, I couldn't miss. I sat on the floor in my T-shirt, parachute pants and sandals, lined up a few speed loaders with .357 rounds in them and put the gun to my head.

2

"But You're Not a Sick Guy."

It wasn't just the disease and what I perceived as my bleak and inevitable disintegration that brought me to such a dramatic moment. It was a month and a half of agony that seemed to come from every direction.

I hadn't been sleeping at all. I was literally a basket case. I felt sorry for myself; for my kids; for my wife; sorry that I even married somebody. I felt worthless, like I'd ruined everybody's life around me. I felt as if I'd ruined my company; I thought I'd probably lose my show. As soon as word got out that I had MS, Paramount would fire me. I didn't know what I was going to do. I hadn't even told my manager, my agent, my lawyer—I told nobody. For the week leading up to my sticking that gun to my head I had set my business in order—making sure I had enough insurance in case I died very quickly.

We had to fly to Los Angeles to tape six more shows on Leeza Gibbons's set—an arrangement we had made months before. All this time I was hurting. My pain had not subsided. On a scale of one to ten, I was fluctuating between eight and ten. It was the worst, most prolonged bout I'd yet experienced, and I was convinced that I was in that 5 percent of people who had the worst type of MS, the one that progresses rapidly until you're trapped in a wheelchair, unable to turn over in bed without assistance, barely able to blink or move your fingers.

My life became a nightmare, both professionally and personally. I had an extremely annoying and aggressive executive producer who was not working out with the rest of the staff, including myself. I had people leaving wanting to claim a hostile work environment. This executive producer would ask me, "What's wrong? What's wrong?" at least sixty-five times a day. I knew she had to be fired and replaced. I also knew that I wasn't the most pleasant person to be around. I became hostile and jaded. I was trying to keep a game face on at work, but I was falling apart inside.

My marriage had begun to show cracks before we went to Utah, and there was little chance they would be cemented after we returned. Grace wanted to star in a movie she and her friend had written—she wanted her life to center more around herself than around me. The timing is never good when a relationship turns sour, but this couldn't have been worse.

I completely shut down. I didn't know what to say to her. I was afraid to be around the children.

I couldn't even think about having sex—my feet hurt so badly; even the attempt to have sex with my wife was more of a chore than any moment of passion could overcome. How could I get my brain to not think about my feet? It didn't matter how sexy, attractive or beautiful she might have seemed—all I could think about, day and night, were my damn feet. And one of the worst aspects was that I didn't feel as if I had the right to complain, so I didn't. I couldn't share this with Grace or anyone else, because no matter how much I explained I knew no one would understand.

And then it got even worse—my skin became hypersensitive. It hurt when I took a shower. If someone touched my arm I'd start to freak out. It was painful if someone walked by me and barely brushed my shoulder. I didn't want people to get that close to me.

For the next three weeks the pain leveled out; it didn't get any worse . . . but it didn't get any better either. Every waking second I knew it was there. Some parts of the day it would lessen; other times it would get worse. I found out what I was experiencing was called neuralgia or "nerve pain."

Each year I have to have a physical for the upcoming season of my show. The studio's insurance dictates it. I didn't know if I should lie to the doctor and not mention that I had been diagnosed with MS or if I should admit it. I decided to let my attorney, Nina Shaw, know what was going on and let her help me come up with a strategy to tell Paramount. In my own mind, it didn't really matter because I had come back from Utah and Boston thinking I'd lose my job, that I wouldn't be doing the show once they found out. How could I pass the physical? How could I be insured?

Hollywood turns on excuses: if you give them one they'll use it. Now I was giving them an excuse to cancel my show. There are very few opportunities for African-Americans in this business to begin with. There have been those who have been trying to knock me off the block for many years. This would give some people a very easy excuse to say, "He can't do the show."

Those first three shows when I got back from Utah took everything I had. My staff must have thought that my acting sojourn had turned me into a jerk. They didn't know that my feet hurt so bad I was not able to concentrate. Every day I had to get up and hide the fact that I was still in the middle of a bout. I was tripping, falling down, bumping into people, knocking things over. What makes *The Montel Williams Show* work is that I'm able to listen and respond to my guests. But I couldn't listen because in between each question I was trying to keep myself from crying. No one on my staff caught it—they just thought I was in a bad mood. I was afraid of everybody who even looked in my direction because I was so afraid that they would pick up that something was wrong with me.

For four years leading up to my diagnosis I was so clumsy that Grace used to joke about it. I would walk down the hallway and bump into the wall. No matter how hard I tried I couldn't keep myself from veering to the left when I walked. I walked in a curve; I still do, though I try to hide it. I hide every symptom that I have very well, but I've grown accustomed to them.

But I wasn't accustomed to them on the night I tried to kill myself. . . .

I was trying to make it look like I was getting my guns in order—cleaning them and putting them away. I had collected these guns over the years—as a hobby, and as protection, to make me feel secure. I had the speed loader lined up so someone would think that I could have just stuck a speed loader in, closed the chamber and hit the trigger by mistake.

Then I lowered it toward my mouth but stopped myself. If I stick this in my mouth and it goes off, that's clear suicide, I thought. My kids wouldn't get the insurance. I had to leave it ambiguous enough that people might think it was an accident. That's why I didn't leave a note. If it just appeared that I was cleaning my guns in my closet and the door was locked so my kids wouldn't come in and then it just went off . . . then it would be questionable and people couldn't definitely call it a suicide.

I had that .357 in my hand for twenty minutes. I had already been in the closet for an hour and a half. I was spinning it around by the trigger—it was a relatively light trigger and I was twirling the gun near my head. Twirling, stopping it, twirling, stopping it. If only the damn thing would go off already. It would really look like an accident because I wouldn't be holding it to my head.

Suddenly I thought, what if I shoot myself in the chest and end up not dying? That would be worse than death.

I sat in one spot playing with that gun for another forty minutes. It hadn't gone off and I began to cry. *I should just climb into bed with the gun and shoot myself, just get it over with.*

I began reassembling the guns on the floor and putting them in their cases, crying all the while. I went into the bathroom and sat on the frame of the big Jacuzzi tub until four a.m., staring at my reflection in the glass shower door. I went into that closet to accomplish something and I didn't do it. I hated myself for not having the guts to end my life. I finally dragged myself into bed and lay there in the dark looking for another idea.

I thought about falling off a tall building. I thought about driving my car into a wall or into the river. At that time I wasn't really driving that much, but I could have driven my car into something. Then I thought: if I drove into a wall or a tree the air bag would go off and I'd probably wind up losing my body and be a head sitting on a shelf; people will keep me alive. Better to throw myself in front of a car than be behind the wheel with an exploding air bag.

I began thinking of where I might "accidentally" fall or trip so I could be run over. I needed to find a place where cars drove fast and couldn't brake easily without getting hit from behind. A circle would be good, and I knew just where one was and it was only four blocks from my office: Columbus Circle at Fifty-ninth Street where Broadway, Eighth Avenue, and Central Park West all intersect. Cars entered fast and traffic flowed. There was no stopping in the middle of Columbus Circle. Especially the way some of those taxi drivers drive. Those guys rarely pay attention to traffic lights or to other cars.

A few days later, after Grace returned, I went into the city to do what I wasn't able to do in my closet. I had my driver drop me at the office on Fifty-fifth Street and walked over to Columbus Circle. This was a good day to die, I thought. I was in a lot of pain. I watched cars enter and exit, waited for the right moment, picked a Cadillac sedan, stepped off the sidewalk and "tripped" on my feet, falling right in the path of that speeding black Caddy.

The driver hit his brakes, swerved around me as I lay in the street, and came screaming and cursing out of his car. "You stupid m%$# f*#$%!" he yelled, and then he recognized me. "Oh, Montel, oh, man, I'm sorry, man. You okay? Damn, man, you hurt?" I couldn't understand how he had missed me; he should have run me over.

He leaned down and helped me up. I was dumbfounded that he was able to stop. I should have picked a damn truck.

"I'm sorry," I mumbled. "I tripped."

He helped me to the sidewalk and I walked back down to the studio to tape another show, still in pain, more depressed than ever.

What a jackass! I couldn't even die! All day I kept rehashing my two failed suicide attempts: how my gun never fired as I twirled it round and round my finger; how that driver missed running me over. I could not believe what a screwup I was. I couldn't do anything right—I couldn't stand without my legs wobbling or buckling; I couldn't walk straight; I couldn't shoot myself; I couldn't get run over.

That night I sat in the den with Grace and said something to her about not being around since I was probably going to die soon.

"And what are your kids going to do?" she said and walked away from me. She spoke not in anger but for the first time in a long time with a sense of empathy, as if she finally understood how much I hurt but wouldn't accept my conclusion and wasn't going to allow me to accept it either.

I began thinking what might have happened if that Cadillac had hit me and just broke my back. I could have wound up in a wheelchair for the rest of my life because of that and not because of MS. And then I remembered a palm reader who once looked at the lines in my hand and told me how I would have some narrow escapes but would live a long life. And I remembered something else as well: that apparition that had come to me months earlier, something I didn't talk much about because people might think me weirder than I already am.

And it struck me as if somebody had hit me in the face with a baseball bat: "How dare you? How dare you!"

I was literally having a conversation with myself: "Who do you think you are? How can you leave behind all that you've got?" I had been so angry that I didn't fall down right. I had spent hours berating myself for not having fallen down in the right damn way. How pathetic! Because truly, no matter which way I might have taken my life, my children were going to suffer. Even if people thought it was an accident. And what if there was something beyond this world? Where do they put those who take their own lives?

That was the day I decided I was going to live, period. That was the day I started to think of MS as a blessing. I had been blessed with so much good fortune in my life. I made it out of a ghetto. I had parents who every step along the way taught me to take responsibility for my actions and to own my decisions. I had a job that paid me millions of dollars a year to do whatever I wanted to do. I had four great children, a big comfortable house in Greenwich, and a forum to speak my mind. I had the opportunities to see the best doctors on the planet. These were all gifts, so why wouldn't MS be another gift?

I thought, okay, Richard Pryor has MS. He's one of the greatest comedians of all time, but Richard's MS in the public eye is tainted. They think whatever it is that's wrong with him is because he free-based cocaine. And Annette Funicello—she had faded from the public eye long before she was diagnosed. I am on television every day. I could be in as many as six million households a day. Maybe that's the reason I have it in the way I have it. People aren't made uncomfortable or embarrassed by watching me, because they can't see the symptoms. They can look at me and say, "Man, that guy's got an illness but he's doing something about it. Maybe we ought to help him."

I sat up all night, my mind racing. I started thinking about all that had happened in the last thirty days. It had all seemed so bad, so dismal, so bleak. What if I turned it around and saw it as a sign? As something that was supposed to happen?

The conversation I began with myself lasted for two days. And when I say conversation, I mean it—speaking out loud. People thought I was crazy! I kept thinking that maybe there is something I'm supposed to get done. When I came home from work the next day, the first thing I did was grab my kids and Grace and spend an hour cuddling with them. If I had found new meaning in my life it had to do with family and work and doing battle with this disease. I wanted to keep my family together to help give me the strength I would need, and though our marriage was on shaky ground I thought that by doing something for Grace, by giving her what she most wanted, it would prove my dedication and commitment. With the kids between us I looked at her and said, "Maybe we should do this movie."

While I had directed smaller things before, public service announcements and promos, this was to be my first feature film. Financed out of my own pocket. I figured it was going to cost me $1.25 million. It was a romantic comedy about three unsatisfied women looking to rediscover the little pieces of themselves that they had given up. The cast included Grace, Cathy Moriarty, Eva LaRue,

Jon Seda, Amy Acton, Daniel Quinn, Daniel Joseph, Tina Louise, and Richard Topol. Besides Moriarty, who had starred opposite Robert De Niro in *Raging Bull*, these were actors who weren't widely known. But that didn't matter to me. I wasn't making this movie for critical acclaim or box-office numbers. I was doing it to keep from throwing myself in front of that speeding truck. And to try to save my marriage.

I hadn't even begun to think about what Grace was going to want if we divorced. I was trying to avoid that bill altogether. That was why I was in preproduction with *Little Pieces*. Grace had cowritten it. Grace was starring in it. I was making it happen for her. We had issues, but I was hoping they could be worked out.

That was the situation when I began preparing for this film. I was coming off two attempts to take my life; my MS was in full-blown flare-up; my wife wanted to leave me; and the contract negotiations with Paramount over the future of my show were coming up. All the literature I'd read about MS said to reduce stress as much as possible and I was turning up all the burners!

I buried myself in the three months of preproduction beginning in the middle of March. I had to interview the first assistant director, the cinematographer, and various other crew members. I went through the whole process trying to hide from everybody that there was anything wrong with me.

I found new friends in Guy Rocourt, my first assistant director, and Albino Marsetti, my director of photography. Together we worked day and night. I confided to them that I had MS. "I can't be stressed out," I said. "I'm going to need decent food; I can't be eating cookies and potato chips." So we got a catering truck. Then we had to find a soundstage, which we did, over in Queens—a huge old-style dance hall with a built-in amplified ceiling that reverberated sound. But it had no air-conditioning.

We began shooting in June and July, right in the dead draining heat of a New York summer. That's when I found out the hard way that heat can exacerbate your symptoms.

I wish a doctor had told me about the heat, but doctors who treat MS don't have MS. No one told me that when it gets hot your symptoms can become more acute or new symptoms may arise.

It was 105 degrees on that soundstage and the heat wreaked havoc on me. I felt fatigued to the point where I thought my brain was going to explode. It was all I could do to keep from passing out. There were times when I would try to get up and take a step, but I would drop to the floor because my ankles hurt so badly. The pain just wouldn't go away. I rented two large air-conditioning units like the ones they use on the sidelines of football games and put them outside that old dance hall. We'd blow some cold air on the set through a big yellow tube for five or ten minutes, then kill it to shoot each scene, and turn it back on after we got the shot. I would sit by one of them to cool my body. I went to the Sharper Image and got one of those little personal air conditioners to bring my body temperature down. I was using alcohol and water compresses. Anything I thought would help.

About three weeks into shooting the heat finally knocked me out. I fell through a table and needed to be carried to the air conditioner. Fortunately, none of the crew or cast saw this.

We worked twelve- and thirteen-hour days. It didn't affect my concentration as long as I was in the director's chair with the air-conditioning blowing. We'd set entire scenes around my chair because I had limited movement. What we told the crew was that I had a severe back injury.

Because of the grueling schedule and the pain I couldn't get to the gym to work out. I was having difficulty moving my left leg. I was also smoking and drinking, far more than I should have been, but my attitude was: Who cares? I'm entitled!

I knew that I had to get attuned to what was going on with my body. If I started losing vision in my eye, I had to stop and calm down. Once I released the stress my vision would return. If my legs were really hurting and getting worse by the hour, then I knew the next day I wouldn't be able to walk. My fear, of course, was that I might become so stressed out that I'd go blind in one eye, or never walk again.

And with the stress of the movie, along with the stress of my relationship—or lack of relationship—with Grace, that was a real possibility.

The heat made the actors and crew grumpy. Actors being actors, some began to show some attitude and get a little pissy. At first, whenever there was a problem, I would be sweet and kind: "Please will you come to the set now. I need to shoot this please. . . ." I'd say "please" three times, bring them all Starbucks coffee—but one day when Guy had helped me out to one of the trailers and put the air conditioner on, I lay down for forty-five minutes because the pain was so bad I couldn't put my feet on the floor. When I returned to the set I began to feel my actors might mutiny. Suddenly I reverted to being a lieutenant commander of the navy. I gave up the pleases and got ugly and mean. "You need to lose your *bleeping* attitude!" I told them. "Clean this shit up!" And they did. They liked being directed.

But my officer act only added to the stress and pain I was feeling. I wasn't on any medication and I really didn't want to take any while working in those often tense, embattled conditions because it clouded my mind. In all the reading I was doing I had come across numerous mentions of how the THC in marijuana alleviated the symptoms of people suffering from migraines, depression, seizures, insomnia, chronic pain, AIDS, asthma, arthritis, epilepsy, glaucoma, pruritus, cancer . . . and MS. This was news to me. I thought of marijuana as something you tried when you were young and had half a day to waste getting high and munching on candy bars, pizza, and Big Macs. The thought of getting high during a workday had never occurred to me. But if any of these findings were true—and there were dozens of books, reports in medical journals, and magazine articles devoted to the subject—then it was worth trying. It would be a miracle to find some relief without chewing on those heavy-duty painkillers like Percocet or Vicodin.

I got a joint from somebody and smoked it. Within minutes, literally, my pain became bearable. I didn't feel the euphoric high that most people do when they smoke; I just felt that I could stand up without buckling, that I could walk without feeling those hot coals under my feet. Believe me, that relief from pain was more exciting to me than anyone's drug high could ever have been.

It was the first time in months that the pain in my legs subsided, and that evening I wanted to celebrate with Grace. Up until this point all I could see ahead of me was a wheelchair and a coffin. Now that this simple joint made my pain subside I felt my immediate future wasn't going to be so dire. I tried to convey to Grace this new outlook. Although we were living together, we had been miles apart. I was wrapped up in all the details of the movie; she was concentrating on her part. Besides my own need to prove I could do it, I was making this movie mostly to appease her and to keep her from leaving. I wanted her to feel good about herself. I knew that she had felt that she was losing her identity being "Montel's wife" and she wanted to regain the spotlight; I didn't blame her for that. While we were shooting, she seemed happy. She was working and fulfilling her dream and that euphoria spread to other parts of her life. My hope was that when it was over we could get back to the business of being husband and wife. But even though she seemed happy, that happiness didn't spill over to the rest of our relationship.

When we wrapped the film, Grace expected that we would just chill out. I couldn't chill out. Somebody had to edit the thing. I didn't want to pay an editor because I was already a few hundred thousand dollars over a budget that would eventually double, so I decided to edit it myself. My fourteen-hour production days jumped to twenty hours in postproduction.

One evening when I got home early enough that she was still awake she said, "I'm not happy." Just like that. Very calmly.

"Not happy with what?" I asked. "The marriage? With us?"

"Yes."

Part of me was angry. I was the one with MS, the one killing himself to produce, direct and edit her pet project, and *she* was unhappy! But mostly I felt shame and defeat. I couldn't make my wife happy. I was unworthy.

"What do you want to do about it?" I asked.

"I don't know."

"That's not a good enough answer; if you're unhappy then you have to make a decision."

She was silent for five excruciating minutes. Then she said, "I think I want a divorce."

On more than one occasion I had told myself it would be so much easier if we just got divorced, but when she said the words I couldn't accept it and be done with it. I suggested we try counseling first and she agreed. But secretly we both knew it wasn't going to change things between us.

As if all of this wasn't enough, while in postproduction we got a call from one of the tabloids saying they had a copy of an MRI I had taken and were going to publish a story about my disease.

"We heard that Montel Williams has MS," the caller said. "We'd like a statement from him. We're not going to take a nonstatement." I had no idea how they got hold of my MRI, but I knew that I had to do something. They called on Friday and were going to press the following Wednesday. My back was to the wall. I had wanted to keep my disease a secret, but that was no longer possible. I called my lawyer and my doctors and told them it was time to hold a press conference on Monday, to preempt the tabloid. That left me the weekend to do what I had dreaded doing since I'd been diagnosed. I had to call my parents and siblings to let them know. And I had to talk to my children.

My mother has always been an optimist. She looks at the world through rose-colored glasses. She can find a diamond in a pile of garbage. If a truck fell out of the sky and destroyed my house, as long as I wasn't in it, she would say, "You know, everything is going to be okay." When you just want to feel good, you talk to my mom. But she had been dealing with some health issues herself, so I'd been protective about adding to her worries. Since I was so unsure about MS I didn't want to cause her any undue grief or anxiety. When I spoke to her, she knew I was upset. I said, "I have something important I have to tell you. I have multiple sclerosis."

My mother's reaction was not surprising. "Everything is going to be all right," she said. "No, Mom," I repeated, "the truth is I'm not going to be all right. I have MS."

My father was also going through stuff, getting ready to retire. He was the first black fire chief of Baltimore and there was a lot of animosity he still had to deal with, even though he had held that position for a very long time. When we talked, it was mostly about work, his or mine. I didn't want to drop my troubles on him, but because of the impending press conference I knew I had to say something. Like my mother, he was also confident and optimistic. He told me about a man who worked with him who for eighteen years battled MS before being diagnosed. Sometimes he came to work with a cane; other times he didn't have it. After he was diagnosed, he started doing better and he didn't use the cane for a year and a half. "You may have it like that," my father said. "Until you find out what it is and how you're going to be, I wouldn't sweat the stupid." That was one of the rare conversations I've had with my dad where he just skipped all the nonsense we often talked about and cut to the chase immediately. I heard what he was saying—worry about it when you figure it out and get past it—and that resonated because at that point in time I hadn't heard of anybody getting better.

When I told my siblings, I just felt their compassion—what do you say when your brother calls you up and says he has a deadly disease? I remember Marjorie was confused, like I was at first, thinking of muscular dystrophy. When I explained the difference, she was relieved! MS didn't seem as bad as what she had been picturing. "Well, you look wonderful," she said. "You look like you're doing fine." Clolita mentioned that she knew some people with MS and I was amazed anew that "we" seemed to be everywhere.

Once the phone calls were out of the way I had to take some deep breaths before facing my children. All four of them were at the Greenwich house at the time and I did my best to hold it together when I sat down with them.

"I'll be honest," I said to them. "I've been to the doctor's a few times in the last couple of months because I haven't been feeling good and the doctor finally explained to me what was making me not feel good." I told them that I had an illness that some people called a disease but that I wasn't going to call it that, mainly because my two younger children didn't know how to handle that word; they were scared of the word *disease*. "It's an illness that's called MS. You're going to be hearing those initials because, you know, Daddy is a public guy because of my show. As soon as people find out that Daddy has MS there's going to be a lot of people who'll have questions, even some of your friends are going to have questions. Their parents will ask them, 'Don't you know this little boy Montel in your school? Well, his dad just got diagnosed with MS; isn't that sad?' And then they are going to come and say your dad is sad. I'm telling you first off: Daddy's not sad.

"On Monday I have to go on television and tell everybody that I have this problem. I don't know what's going to happen on Tuesday but if anybody comes to you guys and asks questions, you tell them you don't know and you send them to me."

Ashley, my fifteen-year-old, was having issues of her own and with me; her response was not to respond. Ten-year-old Maressa started crying, which made me cry as well. My baby, Wyntergrace, was only four. She just got that her daddy was sick. "I feel bad for you, Daddy," she said, and gave me a hug.

Gooch, which is my nickname for Montel, was five and full of questions. "Daddy, are you gonna die?" was his first.

"I'm not going to die."

"What does it feel like?" If I wasn't going to die was I going to be coughing and sneezing? Would my head get hot? My stomach ache? Would I feel like throwing up?

I didn't want to talk to them about the pain. "Right now I have a balance problem. If I close my eyes I lose my balance. I can touch my toes if I hold my head up but if I tilt my head down I fall over. It's because my inner ear is affected by a spot in my brain. I just need to focus real hard so I won't fall over.

"The big problem is the heat; in the summer I can't go outside and go running with you. I'll still take you to the beach but I'm not going to be able to play as much. I'll have to sit underneath the umbrella because the heat just takes it out of me."

At that point I hadn't started any drug therapy but I told them I'd eventually have to start taking medication to help my immune system combat the illness and it would probably be a shot once or twice a day. Like most kids, they got all freaked out about needles, but once again Gooch had a question.

"What's an immune system?"

"It's as if I have an army inside of my body that fights anything bad, like germs, that comes my way. When it sees bad stuff it starts fighting it and most of the time it takes that bad stuff out. But for some reason my army is confused; it thinks some of the good things in me are bad guys and is attacking me."

"Well, why don't you just fire them?"

"I wish I could, but it's like I'm trying to call and they won't answer the telephone. You know how sometimes when you try to call me and Dad's out on the road and can't answer the phone. Eventually I call you back, but unfortunately my army is not calling me back. So I'm seeing doctors who are trying to help get the army to stop."

For the rest of the weekend Gooch asked me a million questions. He really wanted me to explain MS down to the smallest minutia.

How do you explain the degeneration of myelin around nerves to a five-year-old? Myelin is the protective coating that allows the nerves to function without interruption. When sections of it are attacked by the body's immune system the nerves can't deliver the proper messages from the brain. Finally I got an idea and picked up the cord to a lamp. I took a knife, scraped some of the insulation off the cord and showed him the copper wire inside. I said, "Inside everyone's body are nerves. Along with your blood and your muscles, your nerves are what make you move, like this wire makes the lamp work. And every nerve has this stuff around it, a plastic coating that protects the nerve. If you scrape off a piece of this coating, in two or three days the wire is going to start to rust, and the light may not work when you turn it on. MS is hurting the stuff around my nerves, which is making them kind of rusty and stopping them from working right."

I partially cut the wire and plugged the lamp in. The light didn't come on. "See, now it's not working. You can jiggle this wire and maybe get it to work. That's what's happening to my body—sometimes light goes through, sometimes it doesn't."

Gooch wasn't scared for me. He would say, "Don't worry, Daddy. I know you're going to help people get a cure for this." Or "God's going to cure us." Or "Somebody gave this to my dad because my dad's going to get the cure."

My son sees me as this action hero. He was always bragging that his dad is in better shape than the other dads. So after all the time I spent trying to explain what MS was and how it was affecting me he still had a question. "Daddy," he said, "how can you have MS when you're not a sick guy?"

3

I'm Not Turning the Other Cheek

Gooch's question was the one I kept asking myself. How could I have gotten MS? I'm not a sick guy. But in thinking back on my life I can remember certain incidents that may have had something to do with it. From what I read about the disease, I probably contracted it when I was a child and it had just lain dormant for all these years.

I was raised in what at the time was a ghetto, Southland Avenue in Cherry Hill, Baltimore. Our kitchen doubled as the living room and the dining room was in the bedroom. When I was sixteen months old I grabbed a pot of boiling water on the stove, spilling it onto my bare chest and legs, leaving permanent scars. It scared my parents, but my mother was a nurse's aide, so she knew what to do. I'm told that I was in the hospital for eight days. My skin was saved, but that was the first true trauma to my body.

When I was four—my youngest daughter's age at the time of my diagnosis—I had what my parents say was rheumatic fever. My temperature reached 104 degrees. At that time no one knew what it was. They called any weird fever rheumatic fever. Some doctors now believe that every person who has MS may have had a high fever at some point in childhood.

When my mom couldn't bring the temperature down after twelve hours, even after packing me in ice, she brought me to the hospital.

This time I was there for two days. The worry was that with such a high fever I could end up with brain damage. There are doctors today who believe that early childhood fever can affect the brain.

I was pretty much known as a child who spent a lot of time either basking in the sun or recuperating in the hospital. I was the kid who ran with a stick in his mouth and poked himself in the back of the throat. I have scars everywhere—my face, back, legs, arms. I'd fall down, cut my chin, split my cheek. Not so much that I was clumsy, but I was into everything. I had a bout of phlebitis from playing football barefoot when I was nine. From junior high on I was an athlete. I broke my wrist when I fell running to catch a pass and my arm got stuck under this other guy's leg. On the track team, I landed on my face in front of the pole-vaulting box. For the first two years of high school I was on the track, basketball and football teams, and though I had my share of injuries, I was a good athlete.

When I was fifteen I got knocked out by one of the older guys when I first started boxing. He was eighteen, so I didn't think much of it. I enjoyed boxing and did it for five years. I got pretty good at it too. In 1976 I won a boxing championship my freshman year at the Naval Academy. I and a couple of other guys who had won our weight classes were scheduled to fight for the national collegiate championships. One day I got into the ring to spar with a cadet named Vince Herda, a light heavyweight who weighed 185. I was about 150. He hit me with a straight right hand. I saw it coming. It was one of those "Oh no!" BANG! moments. Caught me right in the jaw. A perfect punch. I just remember going black. I didn't hit the floor. I was floating as if I were holding on to a pole but what I was doing was holding on to his arm as he was trying to shake me loose. I heard the referee in front of me, counting, ". . . six, seven . . ." I was like, wait a minute—where were one, two, three, four, five? I was gone for like thirty seconds. I just wasn't lying down; but he knew I was out, so he started counting me down.

In twenty-two amateur bouts, I won twenty-one—and had one draw—and seventeen of them were amateur knockouts. In all those fights, no one ever really hit me like I had hit other people, and Vince Herda hit me harder than I had ever hit anybody else—my heart literally left the game that day. I went back to my room at the academy marveling at how I had just lost thirty seconds of my life.

Two weeks later we were getting ready to go to the East Coast semifinals. I went out running along the seawall of the Naval Academy and I hit a rock. I went down and tore the meniscus of my left knee. One full surgery later (and this was in the days before arthroscopic surgery was common), I was in a cast for nine months. That ended my boxing career.

Before I entered the Naval Academy I was in the marines. Went in right after high school. Not a person in my world thought I'd go into the service, let alone the marine corps, but my parents had already put three kids through college and on my father's salary as a fireman and my mother's as a factory technician they couldn't afford to pay for a fourth. My father had a friend who was a merchant marine— he only worked seven months a year; the other five he was off. The one time I saw him he had on this great suit and jewelry, wore smooth sunglasses, and was making $70,000 to $90,000 a year (back in 1973!) just running tankers from the Middle East to the United States. He'd come home and drink his money away, party with women, go back to sea and do it again. I was impressed and thought of going into the merchant marine myself, but then I spoke to a friend of my brother's who was in the marines and he told me about how he was going to go to college on the GI bill, so I joined the marines.

I took the full battery of medical exams and somehow made it through boot camp at Parris Island in South Carolina. It was tough in those days, before congressional investigations put a stop to the way we grunts were treated. A month before I got there a kid had laid his head on a railroad track and killed himself. I managed to survive with only a scar under my eye from a drill instructor's poking me in my face.

After leaving Parris Island I flew to Los Angeles and then took a three-hour bus ride to 29 Palms in the Mojave Desert, which is in the middle of nowhere. It was only the second time I had been on an airplane. The Mojave Desert is not fun. You've got to put sand covers over your bed inside the building because the sand finds its way into every crack and would completely cover everything. In spite of the extreme heat I managed to run a hundred miles each week. I was boxing and doing martial arts, and someone suggested I weight train. I went to the gym with this weight lifter and did some really bad versions of a butterfly without knowing it. I wound up stretching and tearing my pec muscle. For the next week and a half I kept running and boxing with my pec muscle bouncing around.

I went to the doctor, who was a first lieutenant just out of med school. My left pec was a little bit bigger than my right. It was swollen. He touched both nipples and went, "Ooh. This is really strange. I've never seen this before."

That freaked me out because I didn't know what was wrong. I told him I had been to the gym and was lifting, but he said weight lifting wouldn't do that.

He decided because of the way my left nipple appeared he wanted to do a needle biopsy. He didn't tell me what he was thinking and I didn't think to question a superior officer.

I was just out of boot camp, new to the marines, and the one thing that had been drummed into me was that you didn't do a thing unless you've been given permission to do it. You didn't even speak. So I did what he told me to do. I went in this back room and a nurse came and stuck a needle right in my nipple, drawing out some fluid. I went back to the barracks. The next morning he called me to his office and said he found something and would have to do a real tissue biopsy.

I thought he was going to just scrape under my nipple and then let me out. Instead I was strapped into a device that pulled my shoulders in toward each other, collapsing my chest into the middle. They put me completely under and inserted drains. When I woke up I said, "What did you do?"

"We think you had a whole series of cancerous cells on both sides," he said. So he had done a limited radical mastectomy. That is, he didn't take lymph nodes out, but he took my nipples off, put them on a tray, took everything else out including muscle tissue, and stuck my nipples back on. In hindsight, this was absolutely asinine because there was nothing in the muscle tissue to begin with, but he did it anyway. And he said, "I think we saved your life."

That's really all that resonated with me for the next three days before they let me out of the hospital: that my life was saved because this doctor had caught cancer. It didn't even register when one of the other doctors came by to check on me and said he knew it was kind of messed up. What did that mean? I didn't give it any mind.

I was told I didn't have to go through chemotherapy—but I was scheduled for radiation, before which I was allowed a brief home leave. I went home to my parents relieved that I was going to live. Everyone was happy—we had dinner and the Lord was thanked because some doctor was smart enough to have saved my life. My mortality had been questioned—at only nineteen. It was almost impossible to fathom. I remember lying there in the recovery room when one of the enlisted men came in and said I was probably one in a million. That a man could get breast cancer and survive. Who knows where he got that stat? He was just talking trash. But I was as dumb as dirt. I literally left the hospital praising this doctor.

Before this happened I had applied to the Naval Academy, and during that two-week period I was home I missed one of my scheduled interviews. When I got back and tried to reschedule, I was told I was not deemed a good candidate because I had missed my appointment. Nobody had told them I was on medical leave. I had to go to the hospital and get them to write a letter saying that I had just found out that I had cancer. That's when the doctor said, "Well, actually . . . you didn't have cancer."

"Then why did you operate on me?"

"Because I thought you did."

I just went berserk. My chest had been cut into and mutilated— and there was nothing wrong with me! Had I not gone back to ask for that letter I would never have known—I would have gone my entire life thinking I had survived breast cancer.

This delinquent, irresponsible doctor had just been trying to make a name for himself and was trying to do so on me! I looked down at my chest. I was thin as a rail. Before he cut into me I was lean and hard as a rock. So as soon as I was able to start lifting weights I went to rehab and began what has been a lifelong journey to reshape my chest. I'm proud to say that I got to the point of being featured in *Muscle Fitness* and *American Health and Fitness* magazines, and unless you look at it very closely you can't see what that doctor did to me, but I know it's there.

Three months after this operation, I passed a full cancer screening—blood tests and X-rays—and made it into the Naval Academy. For the next four years, other than one accident that messed up my knee, I was fine. I was physically fit, mentally sharp, and ready to go to the marine corps air, designated as a pilot, and was dreaming of being the first black astronaut. Then a month prior to graduation, just before finals of my senior year, I was sideswiped by yet another medical mistake.

The graduating class had to go for routine precommissioning immunizations. I was in line with 150 others, and every single one of us started to bleed when we got our typhoid/diphtheria shot. Finally someone realized that the injection gun wasn't calibrated properly and was injecting too large a dosage.

Three hours after that shot I had diarrhea, was throwing up and had severe flu symptoms. I was so dehydrated they took me down to the hospital and kept an eye on me for two days. They put me on an antibiotic and it all calmed down. One of my classmates who got sick never went back to the academy. (I was later told there was another person who became an epileptic after that shot, but I can't get confirmation from the military.) So right before graduation I wound up in the hospital and I couldn't take my final exams.

They told me I'd be okay; I was just one of those people who had a severe reaction to the shot. One doctor actually said, "You're lucky." I was so lucky that when I woke up one morning and looked in the mirror I couldn't see the left side of my face. I had gone blind in my left eye.

If you set my life to music, here's where you'd want a big ominous duh duh duh DUH! In retrospect that's when everything that would lead to my being diagnosed with MS started. The typhoid/diphtheria shot had possibly triggered the eye problem, or maybe it was coincidental and my MS would have started anyway. No matter what the true catalyst was, from that point forward, every two years I had a bout of what I now know was multiple sclerosis.

I remember distinctly standing at the sink, looking at my face. Hmm, I thought, I must have slept on something and there's something in my eye. I opened the medicine cabinet and reached for the Visine; it slipped out of my fingers. My fingers were really numb. I tried to snap my fingers and I couldn't. The numbness lasted for about twenty minutes and then went away. I thought: No big deal, I just woke up. My left big toe also felt a little weird, but how much thought are you going to give your toe?

After five days I finally had to go back to the Naval Academy hospital, where they puzzled over my eyes. I had an enlarged scotoma, the hole in the vision in my left eye; a nystagmus, which is a twitching of the eye; and some sort of weeping on my retina that they couldn't figure out.

At this point one of the doctors mentioned something about this weird disease, MS, but then said that I couldn't have MS because I was in much too good a shape. I was ripped: I weighed 190 pounds; I had a twenty-eight-inch waist, with eighteen-inch biceps. So for the next twenty years that was my problem and my blessing. Why? Because that was the same thing every doctor for the next twenty years said: "Look at you—you don't have MS." On the one hand, maybe I'd be better off if I'd been diagnosed sooner; on the other hand, I don't know if I'd be here today if I believed twenty years ago that I had MS. I probably wouldn't be. I would have seen it as a limiting force, as most people do.

Still, at this point I knew there was something seriously wrong, and I was devastated. My vision was considered NPQ, Not Physically Qualified, to be commissioned in the navy. I had been in the service for six years. I'd just spent four years busting my butt to get a commission and they wouldn't give me one. I was the first person in my family to be an officer. I had a cousin who went to Vietnam and he ended up committing suicide. It wasn't like all hope rested on me, but I had an entire family running around telling people I was about to become a commissioned officer and suddenly I was told that I wouldn't even be able to graduate.

Meanwhile the search for a diagnosis continued. Retinal bleeding? Ocular degeneration? A tumor? My parents came and took me up to Johns Hopkins because my mother had a very rare eye disease, similar to glaucoma, and they thought that's what I maybe had. Johns Hopkins said no, it wasn't that, but there was something really odd there that they couldn't figure out.

Next I lost my color vision. I was suddenly color-blind, able to see only browns and gray, until I saw Grace's eyes eighteen years later when my color vision mysteriously returned, probably as a result of a sclerosis shifting on a nerve. No one could figure out what the hell was wrong with me; they just kept sending me to the next doctor's office. Some doctors didn't believe me—they thought it was in my head. I even had a series of doctors who said I was a malingerer—a faker.

I would bark, "I can't tell you why I can't see, but it's not my problem—it's yours." As a midshipman I had no right to talk to lieutenant commanders that way. But I wanted to be very clear—just *look in my eye!* It was fluttering like film caught in a shutter. There was no way I could have been faking.

They put me on a six-month medical hold and began muttering about sending me to Cedars-Sinai in Los Angeles. But to go outside the military system took months of paperwork. Meanwhile I made up my finals and met all the requirements to graduate. I just didn't know if I would ever be commissioned.

Graduation ceremony was what you lived for: to throw your cap in the air and have them take off your first class midshipmen shoulder boards and replace them with ensign shoulder boards. I graduated, threw my hat in the air, but my boards stayed the same. A commission is usually automatic upon graduation, but the navy said it didn't have a job for me. Come on, there had to be a job where I didn't need both eyes! But it was a flat-out no.

I was in this weird medical limbo. They didn't even know what the hell to pay me. The rank of midshipman only lasted until graduation day—there's no such thing as a midshipman in the military unless it's during time of war. I kept getting reevaluated. They assigned me to the navy show band at the academy because while a midshipman I had been in charge of booking midshipman bands into local colleges and schools and for Naval Academy dances. So while they tried to figure out where to put me or decide if they were just going to give me a medical discharge, I went on the road for three months performing in Cleveland, Boston, and other cities. I lived at my sister's house. I didn't have anybody to check in with or out from. At the end of July 1980, my eye spontaneously started to get better. Although I didn't know it, this isn't that unusual when it comes to MS. But every time it goes away it can leave you with some degradation. In my case it left the vision in my left eye no greater than 20/60 with a blind spot that's never gone away. Before this incident, I had perfect 20/20 vision and had been accepted to go to flight school to become a pilot upon graduating from the Naval Academy.

For the marine corps air you needed to have correctable 20/20 vision, that is, 20/20 with eyeglasses. My vision was not correctable. There was nothing you could do about the hole. So I couldn't be commissioned as a pilot. The only places I could go in the navy were certain jobs with limited physical requirements. The only two jobs available were supply corps and intelligence. Okay, I'm not the supply corps type. And within intelligence the only thing available to me was cryptology. I had taken Chinese at the Naval Academy as an elective, so they thought I was commissionable in cryptology. I petitioned the navy to be commissioned. I started that process and it ended up having to go all the way to Congresswoman Barbara Mikulski. Over the course of the next few months from September until the end of November the navy went back and forth on whether they were going to give me my commission. On November 29 I got it.

I was sent to cryptologic training in Florida, and after that they shipped me to Guam for two years. Guam is one of the largest islands in the Mariana chain, an atoll in the middle of the Pacific. It was devastated by the Japanese in World War II. We have two major naval bases there and most of the inhabitants are American soldiers. I continued my bodybuilding training and became the naval communications station physical fitness coordinator, meaning I would administer the physical fitness test to anywhere from ten to twenty troops a day. So every morning I was running between three and four and a half miles. While there I began having weird shooting pains in my feet that would last for four or five days and then stop. I saw both a neurologist and a psychiatrist on Guam, but they were unable to do anything more than fatten my medical file.

Because I was a cryptologic direct support officer, part of my job was to provide on-scene cryptologic analysis, which means I would have to take a team of highly qualified analysts on board a ship to intercept, translate, and analyze the enemy's communications and radar systems. I knew that to advance in my career specialty I needed to go to sea. In May 1981 I went to sea as a cryptological officer, on board the USS *Kitty Hawk* and then the USS *Halsey* in the Indian Ocean. The *Halsey* was providing intelligence to the national data bank on air traffic control. We were able to provide data crucial to identifying two Libyan fighter aircraft that had crossed the "line of death," making an aggressive move toward one of our aircraft, and we shot them both down.

After my deployment to the Indian Ocean, I spent a year studying Russian at the Defense Language Institute in Monterey, California. Of course, my first deployment after a year of studying Russian was in Central America. That, I could never figure out. Once back from Grenada, I went underwater, beginning a three-year tour of submarine cryptologic direct support duty. This was supposed to be the fast track for hotshots and that's where I thought I belonged. It never occurred to me that every submarine I was on was nuclear and that might become a hazard to my health, especially since I worked out every day with weights right next to the nuclear reactor.

On all three submarines I was on, I had to get permission from the captain to bring dumbbells on board. Water is a powerful conductor of sound, so you never want to make loud noises on a submarine. The sound of a falling dumbbell would travel through the water up to 100,000 yards—160,000 yards if you drop it hard enough. And since we were in harm's way a lot of the time—in the North Atlantic, in the North Sea—I had to be very careful with those weights. On all three boats I had a padded locker to store them and I supervised who got to use them. If you made noise even one time you didn't get to use them for the rest of the trip because I wasn't going to let anyone rob me of my privilege of using my weights.

Each tour was anywhere from eighty-two days to ninety-five days hatch-to-hatch—that's the navy term for the time between when the hatch is closed behind you and when they open it upon your return. Every one of those days I worked out in my spare time, which was at least one hour a day. I was lifting weights, doing crunches, and doing push-ups right next to the oxygen generator, which is a fission reactor.

All during those tours I repeatedly lost vision in my left eye. It would go away for two days and come back—and I never said anything about it. But there was worse. After each tour everyone on a nuclear sub gets tested for radiation. On my last tour I was tested for the amount of radiation in my body; it turned out to be four times the standard level. The technician said that the dosimeter was obviously on the fritz and suggested we write down the regular numbers on my chart; it would save a lot of people headaches. I agreed, thinking nothing of it—I felt fine. When I think about that now, it gives me the willies. Who knows if that radiation exacerbated my symptoms?

Of all the ailments and medical mysteries along the road to multiple sclerosis, the single most terrifying occurred ten months before my diagnosis. This was when my enlarged blood vessel caused the month of nose bleeding that led to my near death and visit from that shrouded apparition.

Those first few months of 1998 were very stressful. True, I had just won an Emmy for my show, but Grace had reached a point in her life where she felt that if she didn't make a move to find work as an actress she would just have to accept being "Montel's wife" and the mother of his children. She wouldn't have forgiven herself, or me, if she didn't give it one last try, so she decided to go to Los Angeles and meet agents.

On top of that, I was the target of a frivolous sexual harassment lawsuit, and though I was completely exonerated it wore me down. By the end of March my nerves were frayed and I wasn't sleeping.

One night around four in the morning I felt something really weird, like a bug was on my lip. I jumped up out of bed thinking something had bitten me. By the time I made it from my bed to the bathroom, about twenty feet, my nose had let loose about a half cup of blood on the floor. When I looked at myself in the mirror I thought I was dying.

I ran and told the nanny that I was going to the emergency room and drove myself there. The doctor looked in my nose with a scope and saw a little nick. "Are you sure you're not exaggerating about the amount of blood?" he asked.

"Look at my shirt!" I said. There was blood all over my shirt, my pants and my underwear. I had just put clothes on after getting out of bed.

He refused to believe it. He put a little gauze up my nose and said, "I think you stuck your finger up there and scratched yourself."

I got back home as dawn was breaking. I cleaned up and left for the city. During my usual workout I had a little drip, but nothing like the night before. I got to the studio at seven a.m., and by seven fifteen, I was screaming for help. My head of security and friend, Joe Pryor, came running in and saw blood pouring out of my nose onto the floor. I felt like someone had shot me right in the middle of my face. I went straight to the hospital.

The doctors again saw the "little nick" and sent me to a specialist. That began a saga that lasted thirty days. I was going to the hospital every few days for two-and-a-half-hour cauterizations to stop the bleeding. The ear, nose and throat specialist Dr. William Portnoy went up in my sinuses and burned everything up there. But the next day I was bleeding again.

Grace and I had planned a trip to the Bahamas to celebrate her birthday, which we somehow managed to do. But as soon as I returned I started bleeding again. It was back to the hospital for more cauterizing and burning. I felt really lost. For the first time in my career I had to cancel shows because of my health. I'd gone to the studio but before I could walk down to the set my nose erupted and I was rushed to Dr. Portnoy's office.

The doctor couldn't understand it. He had ruled out the possibility of a tumor but didn't know what the heck the problem was. He recommended a procedure called tamponade, in which a thick gauze pad, shaped like an emery board, is stuffed into the nasal cavity and then injected with saline solution.

"It's going to hurt, so hold still," he warned me.

Even with a numbing agent, I've never felt anything more excruciating. I screamed so loud that it brought tears to even Big Joe's eyes. I held on to the arm of a chair so tightly I almost broke it. A friend of mine, Carol Chartrand, had gone with me for support and I bruised her hands because I held them so tightly.

I left the doctor's office and that night decided to sleep in my studio because I just wasn't up for the ride to Connecticut. To insert the tamponade Dr. Portnoy had used a numbing agent that made me very dizzy. I remember standing in my dressing room and thanking Carol for coming with me; then I passed out. I fell right through a glass table. A glass shard punctured Carol's leg. An hour later, the doctor made a house call. He took care of my cuts and scheduled me for a two-hour cauterization the next morning. That kept me dry for four days. Then I started bleeding again.

I was back in Dr. Portnoy's office at four a.m. He packed my face with gauze and told me to stay in bed all day to let it heal. It was the weekend and Grace had just gotten back from L.A. We were having a good talk about our relationship and whether it was worth saving; just as we were getting ready to have sex, I started bleeding.

I tried calling Dr. Portnoy but he was unavailable, so I called a doctor friend of mine. She recommended an ear, nose and throat specialist in New Jersey, just across the George Washington Bridge. On the phone this doctor said, "If you come to my office right now I will go up inside your cheek. There're blood vessels right behind the corner of your eye socket; I can clamp two off and that will stop this."

"Wait a minute," I said. "You've never seen me and you're going to punch a hole in my jaw? I don't think so."

I decided to call Dr. Portnoy's backup doctor, Dr. Pincus, who probably saved my life. Had I gone to that New Jersey doctor I might have bled out completely through my face or died on his operating table from a heart attack. At least, that's what other doctors have told me. And my kids would have to say that their daddy died from a nosebleed and wonder how that could have happened.

Blood was still pouring out of my nose when I saw Dr. Pincus, who put me in an emergency care unit. He told me he suspected an unusual malady that affected 1 in every 400,000 people, a congenital condition that caused the veins in my sinus cavity to grow larger than their normal size. Mine was probably exacerbated by two broken noses in my boxing days. The treatment was to put a balloon up the sinus cavity and pump it full of air, which put pressure on the base of the brain and would hopefully stop the blood flow. It was as excruciating as the tamponade, but this time it seemed to stop the bleeding.

They placed me in the ICU and then we discussed my options. Dr. Pincus was certain that an enlarged blood vessel was causing the bleeding. He described a procedure in which a team of doctors would insert a tiny screen into the blood vessel, then blow small particles of plastic alcohol-based resin against the screen to form a permanent barrier. The idea was that new vessels of the proper size would sprout at the site and supply the sinuses with a proper blood flow. The only problem was that if even one of those particles went past the screen, it could go to the brain and cause a stroke. I could become paralyzed or unable to speak . . . or die.

"What are the chances that might happen?" I asked.

"About fifty-fifty," the doctor answered.

"What?"

I wasn't ready for such a high-risk operation. Instead they took an X-ray and did an MRI, confirming that there was no tumor. What they did see was that the blood vessel leading to my sinuses was about as big as a regular drinking straw when it should have been the size of a cocktail straw. I felt I had no other choice but to risk the operation.

I signed the papers to allow the surgery. A few minutes later I felt a squirt of blood shoot out my nose.

That's when I saw the monitor go to zero and was visited by my guardian angel, who told me, in no uncertain language, to "calm the #@*%! down." It was, no doubt about it, an out-of-body experience. And it put me at peace with myself, in spite of the fact that I was about to go through a twelve-hour operation.

The surgery was a success. After forty days I had finally stopped bleeding. I was in the hospital for five days, and when they discharged me I realized that I had one new fear, and that was of hospitals themselves. Every time I saw the H sign, for Hospital, I thought of death. Death was a very prominent part of my life for a while. I had a fear of death before that experience but it changed afterward. My whole concept of death changed that day when someone or something came to me and told me I still had miles to go before I slept. But it didn't alter how I felt about hospitals. They weren't places I wanted to visit anymore.

For more than twenty years I had seen doctors for serious health problems no fewer than thirty times. I saw fifteen different military doctors, including four military neurologists, and fifteen civilian doctors. Only two of them thought I should be tested for MS and I talked them out of it.

I reflect back on my life and I see that I shocked my body and probably my nervous system when I poured boiling water on myself as a toddler. I was in the hospital with a 104-degree fever for eight days when I was four years old. I was knocked out completely when I was fifteen and knocked down for the count when I was twenty. As a marine I was misdiagnosed for breast cancer and operated on. At the Naval Academy I was given a typhoid/diphtheria immunization overdose, and lost the vision in my left eye. My vision problem persisted while I worked out next to the nuclear reactors on three submarines, exposing myself to excessive radiation. A vein burst in my sinus cavity and I nearly bled to death; before the operation to correct it, I flatlined and came back to life.

How much of all this caused stress to my system and perhaps

triggered whatever it is in my body that makes my white blood cells attack the myelin protecting my central nervous system I can't tell you, and neither can any of my doctors. It's a weird mother of a disease, this MS. It takes a lot out of me. But you know me. I'm a fighter. I'm doing the best I can to keep it under control. I've often said that MS got the wrong guy when it came into my body because I'm not going to take it lying down. I'm not going softly into that good night. I've been motivated all my life to prove people wrong and this invasion within me only makes me think about the slights and hurts I had to go through growing up. I had a few slaps to my dignity that I've never forgotten—and I've grown a lot because of them. I've never turned the other cheek and let something pass; that's not my style. I'm not turning the other cheek this time either.

4

"You People"

I've never been able to get around the phrase "you people" when it comes to color. There's just something about those two words that brings out the soldier in me. And by that I mean the soldier who has been trained to stand up and defend himself against all enemies, ready to take on verbal as well as physical assaults. This happened most recently in Los Angeles at the Annual Nancy Davis "Race to Erase" MS fund-raiser, of which I was one of the honorees and the auctioneer.

One of the items in the silent auction was a beautiful woman's watch covered with pink diamonds. The list price was $16,000 and the opening bid was $4,000. Someone had signed the sheet at the low bid and someone else had raised it by the minimum $100. A third person had jumped it to $4,300. I had someone special in mind, so I decided to up the bid to $6,000 and put an end to it. An hour later I returned to where the watch was on display, looked at the bid sheet, and saw that I was still the top bidder. Then this well-dressed woman came by, eyed the watch she was obviously interested in, put her arm around me, and said, "So, Denzel, are you hawking over my watch?"

I was offended. Had my picture not been in the program, had I not been one of the event's honorees, perhaps I would have taken being mistaken for Denzel Washington as a compliment. Instead, I got angry.

I shrugged her off. "I don't see your name on this watch, and since you don't get names right anyway I seem to have the top bid."

She looked at me confused, so I added, "And by the way, I'm not Denzel."

She leaned over and said, "Oh, geez, I'm sorry—you guys kind of..."

Kind of what? All look alike? As soon as she said "you guys," I heard "you people" and I was done. It was no longer about a stupid watch; it was about me not being just another black man in someone's way.

"You know what?" I said. "I don't know you, you don't know me, and I don't think we really need to be talking." I moved away from her.

"Oh, you don't have to be offended," she protested.

"Well, I am offended, so I think we ought to let it go."

But she couldn't let this go. She had to get the last word in or make me believe she wasn't the racist that she was. "Well, I don't understand why you are so upset about this because it was just a mistake."

"You said, 'you guys.'"

"I didn't mean it that way. . . ."

I didn't want to argue with her. I held up the watch and said, "Is this the watch you want?"

"Yes."

"Well, guess what, you're not getting it."

She gave me a hard look and left. Five minutes later her husband appeared. He tried to make light of the situation. "Ho ho ho, are you the guy who's trying to get this watch from my wife?"

"Let me tell you right now, your wife's not getting this watch."

He shrugged and said, "Ah, man, you probably have a million watches."

"Yeah, I probably do, and I don't care if I had sixteen million watches, I'm getting this watch."

There was one minute left in the silent auction. He looked at me and I looked at him. "Dude," I said, "don't be ignorant. I've been standing here at this table waiting to get this watch. There's one minute to go and you think you're going to add a hundred bucks and outbid me?"

He bent over and wrote $6,200 on the bid sheet. Before I could raise him, time ran out. In such a situation there is one last silent bid, where each of us was allowed to write a number on a piece of paper and the watch would go to the highest bidder. I figured he was good for another couple of hundred dollars, so I just doubled it and wrote $7,000.

I gave the watch to a former girlfriend.

Why did it come to that? Because of "you people." It just brought back bad memories.

I was one of "you people" to the white folks of Linthicum, the community in Anne Arundel County where I and a handful of other people of color were bussed. Of course being six years old, I didn't know that then, but I caught on real fast. As soon as I got off the bus on my first day of school, I saw these good white people, many of them parents of children attending my new school, with their hand-printed signs jerking up and down above their angry faces. I was still learning to read but these signs didn't have many words. They all said the same thing, and they were very clear: "Niggers Go Home!" And in case I didn't see the signs, they made sure I heard what they said. "Nigger" was shouted like it was a curse word. Those who didn't have signs waved sticks at us—all three or four of us black students who had come to integrate their children's school.

It scared the hell out of me. I grew up in an America where people were shooting at integrated elementary schools and burning crosses on front yards, and now here were all these angry people directing their attention at me. Their world was in danger of crumbling all because the color of my skin was different from theirs.

And when John F. Kennedy got shot in the head a year later, I feared that's what these people might do to us when we got off the bus. All through the second grade I feared for my life. These details remain as vivid in my mind as a motion picture. I had this fear of going to school every day. I worried about not being good enough.

I have to give my father some credit here, because in his anger about his world he had wise things to say to us children. He had integrated the Baltimore City Fire Department and lived through unbelievable racial hardships. He wanted his children to have a better life. Though he was strict and had high expectations of us, to this day he doesn't recognize how much of what he said reverberated inside of me. One day when I came home and told him about the signs and the shouting, he said: "The man's gonna look at you as a nigga, but it's up to you to be one."

Thus I learned that I had a responsibility to define myself. If everyone was going to look at me all the time, then I might as well do things that made being looked at worthwhile. And that meant I'd have to excel, even if doing better than most of the white kids in my class pissed off a lot of my teachers. Which it most certainly did.

One of the biggest motivating factors in my life stems from when I was eight and in the third grade. I used to write these stories in school and a couple of them were read on the local radio and printed in the local newspaper. Well, this one story I wrote was about buying Christmas presents for my parents. I didn't have enough money for wrapping paper, so the store owner said if I cleaned up the back of her store she would wrap them for me. I did and she wrapped the gifts. Until this assignment I had never received anything below an A. This teacher, who I knew never liked me anyway, put a big F on my paper and circled one word each time I had used it, all the way around the paper. After class I took the paper to her. I couldn't understand what was wrong. I thought it was a good story.

I asked why I got an F and she said, "Because you people have only one thing on your mind and that's why you'll never be nothin' in your life."

I folded up the story and hid it from my parents. I hid that piece of paper under my mattress until the fifth grade, which was when we started learning to use a dictionary. I looked up the word that was so wrong and discovered that I had misspelled "wrapped." I had put "raped." This teacher had actually looked at me, an eight-year-old, and said, "Because you people have only one thing on your mind and that's why you'll never be nothin' in your life." That experience has become part of who I am. From that point forward I was going to prove that woman wrong. It gave me an insatiable drive.

But I have to admit—it's disturbed me my whole life. It's part of the reason I work with kids. I could have gone the other way. I could have lived down to her sick expectation; I could have been what she thought I was supposed to be. It took me almost forty years and a lot of therapy to finally get beyond it. When I told my therapist about it she said, "Montel, you need to pity that woman."

I look back at my African-American peers and friends who went to that same school and a lot of them never even made it out of the neighborhood. Every day after school a bunch of us around the same age played basketball and talked about things that had nothing to do with school, because we were looking for relief from all the tension we felt. Some of the other kids responded to what was happening to us by ignoring it. Some did by fighting. Several of them are dead now.

It will probably take generations for historians to measure the impact forced integration had on us. But I know what it did to me. It made me a fighter. Walking through a gauntlet of enraged adults hollering about killing blacks had a lasting effect on me. Having a teacher tell me I was never going to be nothin' in life had a lasting effect. I don't care what any sociologist says. I know that faced with these circumstances, you're going to do one of two things. Either you are going to live down to the expectations and become worthless or you are going to fight forever to be somebody, even if it means lashing out. That's what I've been doing all my life.

I'm the way I am because I've constantly been trying to prove those who classify me as "you people" wrong. Because "you people" will never amount to anything.

I know I am a black man every minute of every day. And in spite of all the obstacles that have been placed before me, either legislated or just through attitude, I know that I'm not going to allow somebody to hold me back. I learned early on, as a child, that no matter what I did, our society was not going to allow me to forget that I'm a black man. Nor do I want them to. In recent years, since I've become a talk show host, I keep running into this issue with a lot of people who want to question whether I know I'm black. Some of them do so just because of the way I articulate my stances on my show; others do it because they know that my two ex-wives were both white. I was eleven when I found out that my mother was half white. That made me realize, being bussed to school and growing up with all kinds of people, that if I hate the girl or boy sitting across from me just because she or he is white, then I hate my mother. And what right do I have to hate my mother? Or to hate myself? So I reconciled a long time ago who I am. And the fact that I don't speak down to some people's expectations and invert some hip-hop Ebonics on my show does not *not* make me a black man. The fact that I could fall in love with somebody because that person loved me for the content of my character and I didn't judge them based on the color of their skin, that also does not *not* make me a black man. I get tired of being evaluated by blacks and whites who say things to me that they would never say to a white talk show host. Whites will marvel at how articulate I am; and blacks will wonder why I don't date any black women, when they have no idea who I've been out with in the last twenty years of my life. I've come a long way from the time I learned that my mother was half white. Before that time I was using all the honky terms, all the nasty cracker terms, in my house only to learn that I was really talking about my mother. I felt guilty but also confused.

But it didn't slow me down. I had too much anger, too much to prove, and a ton of self-doubt to overcome. So I became an overachiever.

In elementary school I drew pictures and got some accolades for them. Some people didn't like the attention I was getting. They made me feel I had to justify my existence. I learned how to navigate around potential situations and that a quick mouth could keep you from getting in quick trouble. So I concentrated on my verbal skills. I started performing in front of audiences in the third grade. I sang at a talent show in the fourth grade. When I was in the fifth grade I sat on the stage on a barrel strumming a bass guitar and singing a bad version of Otis Redding's "Sitting on the Dock of the Bay." I started public speaking in the seventh grade. I entered student politics and became the president of my junior and senior classes. I acted in school plays, played sports—all the time learning how to respond to people looking at me.

When I was still in the ninth grade I started performing in a band as the lead singer. We played in nightclubs and I had to act older. I got so good at it I could convince women five years older that I was capable of doing what twenty-year-olds of the opposite sex do. The other guys in the band, all in their twenties, got a big kick out of my losing my virginity so young. The guys all deferred to me, allowing me to negotiate our contracts and set up playing dates.

You better believe I practiced some swagger when at age sixteen I had to walk into a lounge and sit down with a genuine mobster who was telling us we had to play a gig for less money because of some piece of paper he claimed we had signed.

"I didn't sign a contract with anybody," I said. "I can't, because I'm a minor. Two hundred dollars is bull. You promised us two hundred fifty. I ain't playing and I don't have a contract. And they're with me."

I was lucky the mobster didn't shoot me, but he paid the extra fifty dollars. I was the *man*. I started arranging to have our band play at school fund-raisers, where we'd split the money with the school. On the student council I'd raise the issue and convince the members to vote yes; then I'd put on my rock 'n' roll hat and put money in our pockets.

I wasn't hearing the "N" word my last few years in high school, but as soon as I got to marine boot camp on Parris Island a priest made sure we "people" knew who we were. It was Christmas morning, 1974, and race riots were occurring in certain areas of the country. Eight hundred of us were listening to the priest's sermon. "Lord, please pray for the niggers who have lost their way and are destructing America this way," he said. The 40 percent of us who were black snapped our heads up, hardly able to believe we'd heard what that white racist pig was saying. I was sick about it. But I was in boot camp. I was lower than dirt; I wasn't entitled to opinions.

So it happened in elementary school. It happened in junior high. It happened in the marine corps. It happened at the Race to Erase fund-raiser. And all it did was make me stronger and more determined to show people who thought that way that they had better open their eyes to the greater truth: that we are all individuals and not "you people." And some of us can climb higher than others if we have the inner drive.

To some, how I act and react spells arrogance.

In boot camp I was named the honor man for my company and was meritoriously promoted to private first class. None of my superiors wanted that to happen. The drill instructors all thought I was too arrogant. It wasn't that I was arrogant, just sure of myself. I wasn't going to cower before any man. We all put our pants on one leg at a time. Every step along my chosen paths I've defied anybody who would hint that I am not their equal, and that has caused issues.

As a private first class in the corps I was troop handler, a position normally given to a corporal or higher. Then I was meritoriously promoted to lance corporal, then corporal, and then sergeant. Six months after boot camp I entered the Naval Academy prep school and then got a presidential appointment to the Naval Academy. Of the forty marines who entered the prep school trying to get to the Naval Academy, only eighteen of us graduated, only eleven of us got appointments to the academy and only four of us graduated from the academy four years later. And only one of us was black.

Yet, and I say this in all honesty, I've never been driven by accomplishment, but rather a sense of not being good enough. And since I've never been good enough, nothing I've ever done has really felt like an accomplishment. A commissioned officer in the navy? Not good enough because I didn't get a Navy Cross. A successful talk show host for thirteen years? Not good enough because other talk show hosts who are white and have only been on for a year or two earn more money. With all that I have achieved and with all the abilities that God has bestowed upon me, I still, at times, think that I'm not living up to my full potential.

There are and have always been times when I felt my back was up against the wall and I wasn't going to be taken down without a fight. When the tabloids let me know they were going to announce to the world that I had MS, I felt they were about to put my career in jeopardy. How could a talk show host talk to people about their problems when he had perhaps an even greater mountain to climb? When this "exposé" was about to hit, I had already won an Emmy and the show's ratings were pretty high. My fear was that my diagnosis, if found out, would provide the excuse for those in the business to deny my success and strip me of my show. Like that third-grade teacher's remark to me, the tabloid's eagerness to break the story was another negative motivator for me. I wasn't ready to let a tabloid determine my fate. As far as I was concerned, when I heard about this on a Friday, I was ready to do battle by Saturday. And on the following Monday, I took the bull by the horns and stepped before TV cameras and print journalists to welcome the world to my coming-out party.

5

If the Mind Believes

On Sunday I called Frank Kelly, who was then senior vice president of Paramount domestic television, and Bobby Gableman, senior vice president for off-network production, syndicated programming. In a voice I tried hard to keep from shaking, I told them I was going to hold a press conference to announce that I had multiple sclerosis. This was tougher than talking to my parents, because we were getting ready to go into contract negotiations and I feared that this was going to work to my disadvantage.

I said to them, "In the last nine months I have not missed a day of work. In the last nine years I have done eighteen hundred shows and only had to cancel one taping." I went on defending my job performance and my value to their company, letting them know that having MS wasn't going to have any impact on my ability to fulfill my contract. That's when Frank Kelly said, "It's not going to have any impact on the way we feel about you. We'll have somebody there standing with you at your press conference."

They asked how I was doing and told me to make sure I told the media that the studio was behind me 100 percent. What a relief! I've never told them this, but that was a huge moment in my life. Instead of rejecting me, instead of getting angry at what this would do to their business, they embraced me, and set my soul at ease. I thought they would say that I was uninsurable and that I was going to lose my job. For them to say instead that they were in my corner and had my back—that was like a gift of longevity, a gift of life. That told me that in spite of this illness I was going to have an opportunity to continue to work and contribute.

On August 23, 1999, in a matter of five brief minutes, I went public with my secret: "I was just diagnosed with MS. Fortunately I'm doing fine. I've been working with doctors here and at Harvard and I'm going to be working very hard to try to raise money and awareness." I didn't go into all the details; I wanted to keep it short and matter-of-fact. But some anger may have crept into my voice when I added, "The only reason I am standing before you is because some paper in this business was going to try and take my private medical records and show them to the world." Then I turned the microphone over to Dr. Olek, who had flown in to answer any technical medical questions.

It was emotional, it was tough; but everyone was respectful and accepting. The New York press has not always been very nice to me, but they were that afternoon. I was anticipating a front-page headline in the *Post* the next day saying something like: *Montel Loses His Job Because of His Illness*. But that didn't happen. Instead they showed a photograph of Grace and me, and you could see the strain in my face.

I wasn't the first celebrity to come down with MS, but because I was in people's living rooms every day it might have been the first time MS had a real face. Certainly the people who watched my show wanted to know more. The next day I received more than 10,000 e-mails, phone calls, and faxes. I was surprised that people would be so supportive. It lifted me up but I was also still waiting for the bomb to drop. That's just the way I've always been, and probably the reason why I'm constantly trying to achieve. But one of those 10,000 messages would change my life.

It was from a woman named Nancy Davis, daughter of billionaire oilman and entrepreneur Marvin Davis (who sold Twentieth Century Fox to Rupert Murdoch in 1985). Nancy was in her early forties and had been living with MS for half her life. She had been through the entire roller-coaster ride. She had gone blind and then had her sight returned; she was unable to walk, and then her mobility returned. In other words, in many ways hers was a typical case of MS. But there was one big difference. She was a wealthy, wealthy woman. She understood money, she was an experienced fund-raiser, and she had started an organization to fight the disease she herself was fighting.

She understood, as I now do, that WE truly are responsible for our medical care, not doctors, not the government. After all, you can ask seven doctors about multiple sclerosis and get seven different answers. You won't find that with cancer or most other diseases—there may be four or five different schools of thought, sure, but everyone basically agrees on where cancer comes from. With MS, everybody has a different opinion. Some think it could be a hereditary disease; others believe it's congenital . . . or vascular or degenerative or psychogenic or toxic or infectious or systemic or viral. There are theories that it comes from insect bites or from canine distemper.

The uncertainty, the lack of research about the disease, was what made Nancy Davis so angry. It was what brought her to found the Center Without Walls, an organization that distributes research funds to some of the top hospitals in the country and brings participating doctors together for quarterly videoconferences and two physical meetings per year, which include a panel discussion that's open to the public. The doctors have to share all data they have gathered with the help of the funds Nancy gives them; if they don't share information they get thrown out of the group. This keeps them from duplicating research and wasting valuable time and money. I don't know anyone else who has been able to orchestrate such a forward-thinking initiative.

Here was this socialite, someone of means, who was suffering from the same illness that I had. She wasn't taking any medication and was doing really well, perhaps because she is a strong believer in personal power when it comes to looking for doctors who would help her chart her own course rather than charting a course that's been outlined by some national organization.

I was curious to see what this woman was all about. If her father was worth billions and she was coming to see me about raising money, then something was wrong with that picture. But that's not what she came to say. She wanted to share with me what she had been going through, having been thrust in the public eye with this disease. She got me to understand that not everything that was written about MS was true. And that's what started me down the path of questioning everything.

She became my new angel, come to help prevent me from going through what she had gone through. We talked about everything: the various fund-raising organizations, the ABC drugs, alternative medication, and about funding research. She had so much information! She had been organizing and funding research for nine years. She had been through the anger and the bitterness of dealing with the disease. I could relate to that.

Nancy had raised two to three million dollars a year for nearly ten years and said that because I had come forward her foundation wanted to give me their Man of Courage award.

I was humbled. My going public was more a preemptive act than an act of courage. I wanted to be ahead of the tabloids and take their fire away from them. If you steal their thunder, you steal their front page. I knew if I held that press conference I would no longer be newsworthy enough for them. I wasn't really deserving of any Man of Courage award.

Nancy waved that aside. "Montel, I'm rich and you're rich. We can afford the doctors and the drugs needed to treat this disease. But there are people out there who cannot afford anything." It was an incongruous picture: this lady sitting in my office with enough bling on to pay for seventy-five people's hospital visits was downright passionate about the downtrodden and the struggling who were afflicted. It was no act. She truly meant what she said. And she knew that no matter how much money she had she couldn't cure this disease by herself.

Then she started in on the pharmaceutical companies and the way the government had ignored the disease. She challenged me to do my own research. "Look at the statistics—they haven't altered in a decade. Don't accept what people tell you, Montel—investigate."

Nancy had very deliberately left me wondering how many people in the United States actually had MS. I went to the National MS Society (NMSS)—and they didn't have the answer. The biggest organization out there ostensibly working to inform people about the disease and raising money to end it, and all they had were some old numbers that they themselves had not verified! The more I looked into the NMSS the more I doubted their effectiveness—and exactly what it was they did with all the money they raised.

Their official estimate was that 250,000 people in the United States had MS. But that seemed ridiculously low. In just the short time since I had been diagnosed, I had personally met dozens of people who had it as well. I had heard from thousands more. Everyone I spoke with mentioned that they knew someone who had MS. And yet the NMSS kept reporting the same 250,000 estimate, for twenty years, which I found appalling. When I asked for an updated estimate of how many people they *really* thought had the disease, they said they weren't sure. If they couldn't give me accurate figures then how could they know who their constituency was?

I was also suspicious because that 250,000 figure would classify MS as an "orphan disease." In legal terms, a disease that affects a quarter of a million people or less is deemed "rare" and drug companies that spend money researching and developing remedies get special tax credits and a minimum of seven years of marketing exclusivity. In other words, any drug company that developed a drug would have a guaranteed monopoly, facing no competition from any other company, for at least seven years. That meant the price of the drugs being developed for the treatment of MS would remain high and that the majority of people who had the disease probably would never be able to afford a cure.

But if the number of people who had MS was in the seven figures, as I suspected, and not the low sixes, then there would be an incentive for more drug companies to develop new drugs to fight the disease. And wouldn't that end up lowering the price of these drugs, because of the nature of competition in the marketplace? This disease does not deserve orphan status. MS should be treated like any other disease that affects a large number of people.

I had another question: How much of the money they raised went to research to find a cure? If you're telling the public you're raising money for a cure, then isn't it simple logic that most of what you raise should go to a cure? I couldn't find the exact percentages, but the NMSS spends somewhere around 30 percent of their operating budget on salaries, while only 20 percent goes to research. That's crazy! We have to stand up and challenge the face of fund-raising across America. Anybody who is raising money to help fight a disease, going and knocking on people's doors and preying on the compassion of the American public, should not be giving *less than half* of what they raise to that cause! I have a real serious problem with that.

After my press conference and my meeting with Nancy Davis, I was obviously pumped to try and do something to further the cause of those of us who were suffering from this disease. With so many people contacting me, offering to make a donation to help find a cure, it seemed logical to look into forming a new foundation, one in which all public donations would be devoted to research. Not 20 percent, 30 percent or even 50 percent—*every* cent. With the help of Drs. Weiner and Olek, I channeled the donations that were coming to me from around the country to a fund set up at Harvard's Brigham and Women's Hospital until my own foundation was properly set up. Within three months they raised $250,000.

But while I put that in motion I had to deal with going to work on the talk show, and I had to continue to work on the postproduction of *Little Pieces*. I had to suffer through the deterioration of my marriage. And I had to confront my oldest daughter, Ashley.

One never knows why a child starts becoming distant and disobedient, but with all the attention in my family focusing on me and my disease, I can almost understand what happened. Ashley was fourteen and like any adolescent was trying to figure out who she was. But she had some special challenges as well. She had finally been diagnosed two years earlier with epilepsy; this came after four very rough years of what we would later find out were miniseizures. A lot of things that should have been paid attention to were not. Ashley was extremely depressed and I didn't see it. I should have but I didn't. It got ugly between Ashley and her mother, so she came to live with us. Then it got ugly between Ashley and Grace's mother. Ashley felt like all the women in her life were down on her. She was angry when nasty things were said about her father, and with my marriage falling apart my home wasn't the happiest of homes. To make things worse, I wasn't always around for her. Sure, I left her in the care of people I loved and trusted, but I should have been there more myself.

Boarding school seemed like it would be good for her, but right away she started partying. We think boarding schools are so supervised and safe, but smart children can get around the rules and regulations. Mine was one of them. Ashley has always been a clever young lady. At the end of the school year, the dean politely suggested Ashley not return. I brought her back to live with me but she spiraled down deeper into her depression. We weren't communicating, so I didn't know—I thought it was a typical fourteen-year-old acting out and I let it go.

I enrolled her in a Greenwich public school and hoped that being at home would be easier for her, but right away she started hanging with bad kids. One of them wrapped a car around a pole on the parkway. Ashley had been cutting school with these kids, and it was only luck she happened not to be there that day. She was suffering from chronic depression from her seizures, and her acting out was so bad it was getting dangerous. I was frantic, desperate to keep her from hurting herself.

I had heard about a disciplinary school in northern Idaho that specialized in straightening out kids who were out of control or who were on that slippery slope toward self-destruction. I spoke to doctors, friends and one of my attorneys. People I trusted told me that this was a legitimate program; they had doctors on staff who could help her handle her medication and her epilepsy. I had my doubts—the school was a total lockdown facility for children with behavioral and emotional issues. I was concerned about Ashley's striking ability to sell anybody. I don't care how many credentials a psychologist might have, Ashley has taken some of the best doctors in the country and turned them into malleable pawns. I was concerned that this might happen again. I was also concerned about Ashley's emotional needs. She was dealing with depression in an unhealthy way. The people at this school were supposed to have the ability to help a child navigate those waters. But would they be able to help her or would she figure out a way to snow them? I thought, at the very least, she'd be in a place where she would stay alive. I'd worry about the other things when we got past that one.

I made the arrangements without letting her know anything. I packed her clothing and medication and hired a couple to come to the house to escort her on a private jet waiting at Greenwich Airport. One morning, at six a.m., I woke her up and told her that her behavior was beyond what I could handle and that I didn't want her to live with me until she realized that some of the things she was doing were dangerous. She cursed me and yelled at me. I didn't want her to see me crack, so I told her that I loved her and that it was a process we had to go through. I walked out of the room an emotional wreck as the couple I'd hired walked in. They put her in a car without incident and took her to the airport.

After she arrived at the school, I didn't speak to her for a month and a half, until the day before Christmas, which was the school's policy. I felt awful. There was a small amount of relief mixed in, but mostly I felt like a horrible, guilty failure. Not only had I failed completely as Ashley's father, but the brave public face I was putting on MS was about to push my marriage over the brink.

People magazine had covered my press conference in a small story, but they had received so many letters about me that they decided to do a follow-up cover story with the headline MONTEL'S TOUGHEST FIGHT. Grace had asked me again for a divorce, but we had decided to try to work on it. Maybe it was because we truly believed we were going to get through our issues and stay together, or maybe we just thought if we talked ourselves into staying together, we would. After all, she couldn't walk out on someone who had just been diagnosed with MS, could she? What neither of us realized was that she had left long before that; she just hadn't physically gone out the door yet.

The day that the magazine came out, with its glossy cover depicting Grace and me in a loving embrace, I was sitting in an editing bay working on this scene in *Little Pieces* where Grace takes this guy up to her room and makes love to him. If that wasn't stressful enough, an assistant came into the bay with that *People*. Two days earlier Grace and I had had a conversation about whether we should start seeing lawyers. We came to no conclusion. Now I was looking at the two of us on the cover and wondering if it might change anything between us.

Besides the cover shot, there was a full-page picture of the two of us inside. She was in my lap, with my arms around her. Above the photo was a quote from me: "Because of the power of my love for this lady, I am going to be back in rare form." In the story they quoted me again: "Gracie's the reason I'm able to get out of bed every morning." And it quoted her: "It's just pure belief and love in this person I know. I know his courage and strength and heart. . . . Montel's . . . just a person who is loved."

Loved all right, but not by the woman who said that. Or at least not loved enough for her to wear the same face in private as she had in public.

When Grace came into the editing bay, I showed her the magazine. We went into a second room to look through it together.

"So," I said, "what are we going to do?"

"I still want a divorce," she said.

"Done." The idyllic couple preparing to do battle together against a potentially debilitating disease was a fantasy, if not an outright lie. It was a nice picture we had painted for *People*, but no matter how much we wanted it to be true, it just wasn't. The power of my love was not enough to keep us together. But the power of my will was determined to keep the disease at bay even if I had to go it alone.

I called Dr. Counter and unburdened myself—about Grace's decision to leave, about sending Ashley away to Idaho, about the financial hole I had dug trying to turn *Little Pieces* into a commercial movie, and about the simple fact that I wasn't well. Where could I possibly get some relief? I certainly never expected his reply: he suggested we take a trip to Sweden.

It seems Dr. Tomas Olsson was the director of the Department of Molecular Medicine at the Karolinska Institute in Stockholm and in charge of their MS neurological department. He did the European clinical trials on Copaxone and Betaseron, two of the MS drugs. Dr. Counter urged me to see him for a more thorough MRI and to have my medication checked to make sure I was on the right path.

I had turned my medical care over to Dr. Counter to manage. He is one of the gentlest, kindest men I have ever met, and I knew—just knew—I could trust him. If he wanted me to go see some doctor in Sweden or India or Kuala Lumpur, I'd go. That he was willing to join me on the trip made me feel all the more secure.

At first Grace agreed to accompany us, but at the last minute she changed her mind. Even though we were emotionally separated, we were still living in the same house and I thought I could count on her for moral support. I should have known better.

I was scared. I was heading into this dark Scandinavian cave with no idea what to expect. Doctors and nurses who didn't speak English were going to wire me up and do all kinds of tests on me and for all I knew I might roll out of there in a wheelchair. Because according to Dr. Counter, I was going to see a wizard. This Dr. Olsson was a genius. I was pretty sure he was going to tell me if I needed a heart, a brain, or some courage to prepare for my impending demise. I was going to accept whatever this genius told me: if he said I was dying, I was dying. After all, 3 to 4 percent of people who have MS die from complications in the first three years after being diagnosed. Maybe he was going to tell me what percentile I was in.

On the long night flight over, Dr. Counter tried to make me feel more comfortable by explaining what I should expect. "This isn't a major thing; it's more like a minor major thing," he said. "Maybe Dr. Olsson will tell you Dr. Olek's plan of action for you might not be the best. Or maybe he'll tell you you're on the right track. The research they're doing on strokes and other abnormalities of the brain is more advanced than what we're doing in the States. Besides, this trip could be a good opportunity to just sit back, clear your head, and chill yourself out."

I didn't know if everything Dr. Counter was telling me was true or if he was just trying to distract me, but I got so engrossed in what he was saying that I began thinking there was hope. I decided I would focus on that hope rather than on dying.

My first visit to the institute was in the evening, after the regular patients had been taken care of. In spite of my aversion to hospitals, this one wasn't anything like the sterile modern hospitals I had grown to loathe. It seemed more like a World War II hospital. European buildings often look like big parking garages and this hospital was no exception. It was stark, dreary, drab, and painted that hospital gray. I saw people on foot scooters scurrying along these mazelike underground corridors to deliver things from one section to another. I remember walking upstairs and wondering what I was getting myself into. I had to smack myself in the head to remind myself that this was one of the leading medical facilities in Europe and that not everything had to be plastic and antiseptic like in America. As old as it seemed, everything was spotless and meticulously clean.

I first saw two prominent doctors: Dr. Börje Bjelke (pronounced Bel-Key), who was in charge of the MRI research, and Dr. Hans Persson, from the Pasteur Institute in France, who ran the Karolinska's brain conductivity and signal analysis department.

The institute's MRI machine looked like something out of a sci-fi movie. In the United States the MRI is a diagnostic tool that identifies scars or lesions. In Sweden, doctors try to look at the lesions individually to see if they're expanding and to see if cells are dying around the lesions, which can help determine whether the disease is active or not.

As in the United States, I was given earphones to soften the noise of the mammoth machine as it spun around me for three and a half hours, registering the magnetic flux through my body. The computerized images would show slices of my brain down to a hundredth of a millimeter.

I studied Dr. Bjelke's face while he examined my MRI and tried to guess what he was thinking. All I knew was that he looked concerned, and that scared me.

Then I went through a conductivity test, which involves a device that cycles from cold to hot very quickly. The technician placed it on different parts of my body; as it went through its temperature cycles, I had to press one button when I felt heat and another when I felt cold. Simple enough, but the test was very unnerving. Parts of my body were so numb that I barely felt anything at all.

Of course, it was Dr. Olsson who had ordered these tests, and when I was done with them the staff took me to see the grand wizard himself, who would pronounce his conclusions.

Dr. Olsson was a very quiet, small man who just needed bigger hair and a mustache to look like Albert Einstein. He is hailed as probably the top MS specialist in Europe—he's certainly the leading contender to identify the gene that could possibly be the trigger to MS—and he makes all of $65,000 a year. It isn't about the money. He is a hero. When we walked down the hall, there were as many people scurrying away as there were people coming to genuflect. Swedes don't revere celebrities the way Americans do, but when you were with him, you knew you were with a celebrity.

He didn't speak to me at first. Instead, he examined me with a needle, touching me and watching my reflexes, my movements, checking my balance. Once his clinical evaluation was done, he began to talk. In his slow, meticulous "Swinglish"—part Swedish, part English—he told me almost everything I could have hoped to hear.

I described everything I was taking: the Vicodins, Percocets and other powerful painkillers; the vitamins, minerals, holistic herbs and injected human growth hormone (HGH). His reaction to everything was considered and thoughtful. He'd say, "Vitamins? I don't know. I look for harder science but vitamins don't hurt—keep doing." He wasn't so sure about the HGH because he'd seen negative results in some people, but that was at twenty times the dosage I was taking (and I knew bodybuilders who took forty times that amount!). "People in Sweden don't take this. I think the person getting the most benefit from it is the person you're paying. But if it helps your physicality at this low dosage, then no harm no foul."

When I asked him whether it was all right for me to work out, he said to do whatever I could physically do, but not to the point of strain. I had to become highly attuned to my body, to know the difference between exhausting myself to the point of absolute fatigue and exhausting myself just enough for minimal weekly gain.

Then we discussed my drug therapy. (I would prefer not to name which ABC drug I take because I don't want people to think I am endorsing it. I can't make the claim that because I am doing well this drug must be completely responsible. I take a three-pronged approach to my medical care: holistic, hormonal and prescriptive. It's expensive and I don't want to single out any one herb, drug or hormone because it's impossible to say what definitively works for me.) I had only taken the ABC drug at this point maybe ten times and Dr. Olek had warned me not to even think about getting any better for three to six months. The reason, I think, most patients are *not* told the truth about drug therapy is that it takes so long for it to start being effective. If you're going to put a big pill in your mouth four times a day or inject a drug daily and the doctor informs you that it's going to take a week or more for it to start working, a lot of people are going to stall for that week before taking them. They forget that you need the other days to get enough of the drug in your system for the drug to start becoming effective. It takes your immune system quite a while to figure out that that stuff floating around in your body is something that it needs to attack. But even though I knew it was too soon to feel the effects, I was still desperate for reassurance that the drug was the right one for me. Dr. Olsson immediately concurred. Because in his expert opinion I clearly had relapsing-remitting MS, he said it was the best thing for me. My reaction was one of major relief. I was looking at a lifetime of sticking this needle into my body every single day and I was glad to have it confirmed that it was something I needed to do.

Dr. Olsson explained the MS "seven-year rule": however you are for seven years will be how you will be for the next seven years. If you've demonstrated any worsening of symptoms over a seven-year period, you'll probably see the same level of worsening or degradation over the next seven. If you stay flat, you'll probably stay flat. If you've had one episode in seven years you will probably have one episode over the next seven years. That's kind of the rule of thumb until you hit a certain age or threshold, and then it seems to be canceled. All of us with MS eventually become progressive, even if we die of something else before it actually manifests itself in symptoms. There are different degrees of progressive, of course; it doesn't mean all of us who have MS will become wheelchair bound. But what this rule of thumb meant to me was a reality check: I may not have as much time left as I would like, but whatever time I had, I was going to live every second to the fullest.

With some hesitancy, I admitted that smoking marijuana reduced my pain. Dr. Olsson wasn't surprised. He confirmed all the information I had been getting about marijuana since the press conference announcing my diagnosis: "I have not seen any quantitative study done appropriately on varied ways to ingest and get that medication in your system—but if some consumption of cannabis is helping block your pain, then I suggest you continue. Because it's better than going down the road of barbiturates or opium-based products."

His manner was so calm and comforting that when he said I was in a pretty good place I wanted to hug him. Here was the most respected man in the business saying to me, "You have MS, but it's not a death sentence." He was the first person of any authority who had said these things to me. For the first time since I had been diagnosed I didn't think I was going to die in a year or be using a wheelchair by Christmas.

I was overcome with emotion when he said that, and I could see that Dr. Olsson wasn't used to seeing grown men cry in his office. To help put my disease in perspective, he told me about a sixty-year-old patient who had so many plaques in his brain he should have been immobilized. He became paralyzed on one side of his body and got over that; then it happened to his other side. He came back from that as well. Then he went blind in one eye, then in both, and within a year he regained his sight. His symptoms just kept reversing and today the man has more problems due to natural aging than to his MS. The way the doctor told me this, in his fractured English, helped turn my thinking around. Why see the glass as half empty when it's really half full?

"You are the same person today as you were the day before you were diagnosed," Dr. Olsson said. "So continue to be that man and we'll deal with the disease as it moves along."

With that, my consultation with Dr. Olsson was over. He shook my hand and said he'd like to test me again in six months. I went back to the hotel with Dr. Counter and bought a Cuban cigar. I felt like a huge weight had been lifted.

We went out for a relaxing dinner; I smoked that cigar and felt, if only at that moment, that I would get through this disease. I started thinking about all the other things in my life that I had gotten through: the tear in my knee, the surgery on my chest, the bleeding through my nose. As silly and clichéd as it sounds, if the mind believes it, you can achieve it—and at that moment I believed it. I believed, I achieved, I overcame. I filled my lungs with that Cuban tobacco smoke and it felt like an elixir that lifted my soul above the ground and allowed me to float.

6

Boxing Pain

Coming back from Sweden I was more cheerful than I had been in months. I thought I was prepared to take on my disease and win. But once I was at home I crashed, like the hangover after an incredible high. I guess subconsciously I had hoped Dr. Olsson would tell me that I didn't really have MS after all, that it was just some central nervous system disorder that would go away and let me return to a normal life. Or if he couldn't tell me that, then perhaps that my MS flare-ups were an aberration and I would soon return to a benign state. Instead I had to accept reality. As nice and direct as Dr. Olsson had been, all he did was reconfirm what that Salt Lake City doctor had told me and Dr. Olek had confirmed. I had to accept the fact that what I had to look forward to was that damn seven-year rule of thumb. The six months of excruciating pain that led to my attempted suicides would one day return. I'd have to face that abyss all over again. Again and again, for as long as I lived.

Instead of returning prepared to do battle, I sank into a deeper depression and sense of hopelessness. For the next seven months I felt like I had joined the living dead.

It was the proverbial vicious circle. MS made me prone to depression, and depression worsened my MS symptoms, which made me more depressed, which made my symptoms worse. . . . MS is a nightmare that way, because the less emotionally stable you are the more it will eat you up. The more you succumb to negative emotions and let them gnaw away at you, the more debilitated you become.

Since I am now prone to depression, I have to pay attention to my emotions all the time. If I feel a depression coming on I have to try to stop myself from going down that path.

Maybe the way other people are affected by the phases of the moon, I'm affected by the flow of this disease in my brain. The depression isn't just about being sad or upset—it's a chemical reaction in my brain in response to the MS. I can be in the midst of eating ice cream and cake, having the best time, or chilling on a mountain for three weeks with no stress at all, and suddenly I spiral down. Unless I can will the brakes on, I can be stuck there for days.

So depression isn't *only* about being sad. But having MS does make me depressed. Why?

I get depressed because my legs and feet hurt. Sometimes the pain is so great that I feel compelled to do something drastic to distract myself from it. I smack myself with a stick, spoon or other metal object—not to dull the pain but to create new pain, which is never as painful as what I'm trying to forget. I've taken a needle and stuck it into my thigh; I stuck one right through my hand to draw blood. I don't know anyone who can really understand this behavior, and when it's at its worst I'm better off by myself, away from people. There are times when I'm crazy, it hurts so bad; I am full of rage. Needless to say it makes me unpleasant to be around.

I get depressed because it is so stressful to manage my anxiety and fear. Walking around all day, holding this in, trying to be strong, makes me start to shake.

I get depressed because my lungs and chest spasm and I feel I can't breathe. It feels like my heart locks up.

I get depressed because my body temperature is completely off. I'm very heat intolerant, which is common among MS patients because heat can exacerbate our symptoms. I feel so hot that I'll get into an outdoor hot/tub only if it is below 28 degrees outside, and even then I'll keep my upper body out of the water. I prefer to be cold. I take tepid showers. I can feel comfortable in a tank top and shorts if it's 4 degrees outside. Yet in the dead of summer I'll sleep with a sheet, a blanket and sometimes a comforter. It sounds contradictory, I know, but I'm just acutely sensitive to temperature changes.

I get depressed because sometimes when I eat I feel like I'm choking. At times I can't eat like a normal person. I have to consciously think about chewing and swallowing every bite.

I get depressed because I sometimes lack balance when I walk. I don't know if I'm going to fall over with each step.

I get depressed because I sometimes get dizzy in the shower or on escalators.

I get depressed because I have vision problems. Sometimes my left eye is blurry. Dr. Olek says my vision can be my thermostat. If I'm exercising and my body overheats, then my vision diminishes and I know I need to cool down for a few minutes. If I'm on the treadmill and I get hot, I have to step off and count to sixty. Then my vision starts to come back. I'll jog for another five minutes or so and it starts to happen again. This has been one of the most difficult adjustments I've had to make. Exercise has been one of the cornerstones of my existence and is even more important to me now. It's my way of reminding myself I'm doing okay.

I get depressed because when I'm sleeping, my body jerks and bounces. I get depressed because sometimes I can't urinate or move my bowels.

Sometimes it gets to the point my stomach and bladder hurt. For the last year I've been running through Metamucil, suppositories, and whatever I can use to go to the bathroom because I just can't go. The nerves in my colon and intestine are not moving waste matter through my body the way they should.

I get depressed because my left hand doesn't work so well anymore. Buttons are my archnemesis. I can't button buttons on my shirtsleeves at all. I've had the buttons taken out of some of my pants and had zippers put in. That's the reason I don't play bass guitar anymore. I've got three basses, and I can't touch them. My fingers are going to have to move faster than they do now for me to be able to play bass. As crazy as this sounds, as soon as I retire from show business, that's exactly what I'm going to do. I'm going to work at it until I can play those guitars again. And the piano, too.

I get depressed because I can't play with my kids the way I used to. My son would love for me to go outside and run with him, but I can't. I can use a Razor scooter but it's hard because my left leg is off balance. I can throw a football and shoot a basketball, but I just can't run enough to play the game. When Gooch throws a ball over my head I can't run backward to catch it. Then there's swimming: when I hit the water the numb spots in my body become even more numb and I can't find my feet at all. I know they're down there but I can't get them to start kicking and paddling. I have to make a concerted effort to think it through.

The only way around it is to repeat the necessary motion over and over again until my brain starts to relearn it. One summer, swimming in Lake Tahoe, I had the damnedest time getting out of the water. My right leg was working okay, but my left leg wouldn't move the way I was telling it to. It took me fifteen minutes to climb out. But the next day I went back in the lake and practiced until I could get out whenever I wanted. Similarly, to be able to ride a bike, I need a full hour practicing in a parking lot, getting my brain to remember the skills.

I get depressed because I don't always know when my penis will get erect, or whether it will function properly when it does. About 85 percent of the time I'm fine, but it's that other 15 percent that can drive me absolutely nuts. I can have an erection and not feel anything. Other times I can walk around all day with a hard-on wishing it would go away. Some men who have MS ejaculate the second they have an erection because they can't control the nerves. Thankfully that's never my issue. Sometimes I can't ejaculate, period. That could be a winner depending on whom I'm with. But it can also be a bummer. And then there have been occasions when I've had to use Viagra because it just wasn't going to happen, period. A lot of men with MS have the same problem. But that doesn't help my self-esteem. It just depresses me.

I get depressed because I have to hide how I really feel. For the longest time after I was diagnosed, my whole existence was about try-ing to hide my pain, not from anybody else, but from me. I just didn't want to deal with it. I thought if I concentrated on any one thing too much it would exacerbate my condition and I would hurt more. So if anyone seemed to be close to guessing how much pain I was in, I would change the subject, talk about yesterday's news, talk about any-thing rather than deal with how I truly felt. Even today if I'm going over potential guests for my show with my staff, or if I'm hanging with friends at a nightclub or restaurant, and I feel that searing pain in my feet, I do my best not to grimace or show how I'm feeling. Sometimes I'll have to excuse myself to let it out in the privacy of a restroom.

There are drugs one can take to fight depression and I've tried many of them, but they don't work for me. Prozac, Zoloft, Paxil. I've seen too many side effects across the board. I tried Zoloft for two and a half weeks but found myself talking to certain friends about committing suicide and immediately stopped taking it. I had my brush with ending my life and had resolved against it. I didn't need a pill that encouraged those thoughts. Some people can take them and need to take them. I just can't.

One of my loved ones is on an antidepressant, and as much good as it does for her, it does the opposite for me. When she doesn't take it she's an entirely different person. Little things throw her off and make her anxious. She can spend twenty minutes sweating some-thing stupid like a look from some woman in a store. When she's taken her pills those looks don't bother her. Me, I'm the opposite.

I'm not going to knock the pharmaceutical companies for creat-ing the stuff. It's just not something for me. I'd rather battle my depression differently.

So, depression comes for many reasons and from many direc-tions, and though I'm aware of how it can affect me I'm not always able to keep it at bay. After seeing Dr. Olsson my spirits were lifted, but it didn't last much longer than the flight back to New York, where I had to face the fact that I would have to adjust my life in ways that I could only begin to imagine.

After Sweden I thought a lot about Dr. Olsson's dismissal of some of the things I was doing, like taking human growth hormone, and his ambivalence toward the holistic and alternative medicines and vitamins. But they felt right to me and I've always believed that we're the ones responsible for our care as much as any doctor.

I expect doctors to give me their informed opinions; then I take those opinions into account while I make my own decision about what course of action to pursue. That's not just my choice but my responsibility and my right. Say I suffer from a disease and want to make my quality of life the best it can be for five years and then die; to me that's preferable to living the next twenty years debilitated so that a dozen people have to take care of me. You may disagree, but frankly it's nobody's business but my own.

Don't get me wrong—I am determined to live as long as possible. The average life expectancy for an African-American male—sixty-seven—is the lowest of any racial group in America. Most doctors say that MS patients have a life expectancy diminished by anywhere from 5 to 12 percent. Because I am a black man with MS, my life expectancy is as low as fifty-nine. But I'm doing everything possible to try and stretch that out. For example, I am convinced that the reason I have so much energy is because of the HGH and the vitamin and mineral supplements I'm taking.

Bodybuilders, weight lifters and athletes who take human growth hormone in large quantities often experience adverse side effects. But taken in low doses, HGH has been shown to help maintain bone and muscle density and there are claims it may help to promote nerve regeneration. Your body manufactures HGH from the time you are an embryo until about the age of twenty-five. From then on, the amount you produce goes down 10 or 12 percent each year, so that by the time you're sixty you're barely producing any. Some scientists believe that if they understood everything about the genetic workings of HGH it would be like the Fountain of Youth; we could actually slow down the aging process. But for now, we do know that it does stimulate cell tissue and repair. Some scientists believe that it may stimulate the myelin regeneration in MS patients. I'm sure it's not a cure, but I figure if MS is damaging my nerves and if HGH can help to regenerate these damaged nerves, then I'm taking it.

To any naysayers, all I can tell you is that I've been on the same vitamin and medication regimen since my diagnosis, and I haven't seen much progression in my MS.

I'm not naive about the "alternative" side of medicine—the illegal steroids, the herbal remedies that range from godsends to snake oil. I took 'roids when I was into bodybuilding twenty years ago, but also more sensible things like creotine, protein, amino acids, and ginseng. So even before MS I'd done a lot of reading about supplements. Now more than ever, knowledge is power. I've learned I need as much iron in my blood as there can be. Ginseng, which increases my energy, and ginkgo biloba, which promotes brain function and memory, I'd take whether I had MS or not.

I read about several other replacement therapy herbs like DHEA, melatonin for sleeping, vitamin E to balance liver and kidney function. I found out about green tea extract, folic acid, zinc, herbs for my joints, naturally occurring brain hormones. I take them all. I'm really trying to prevent atrophy or any signs of not being able to concentrate or lose motor skills.

After I went public I heard from so many people touting cures, from bee stings to flaxseed oil, from chemotherapy to a full lobotomy. One idiot doctor tried to interest me in a "lesion scrape"—he claimed he could go up inside my brain and remove lesions. Some of these "cures" may work for some people, but they seem a bit extreme, even to me. I prefer to stick with the vitamins, minerals, and herbs that I've been taking without any adverse effects.

I take forty pills a day. I've had people tell me flat-out that I'm stupid. Others have said, well, it couldn't hurt; but they don't really believe it can help.

My response is simple: if I go away for two days and forget to pack my vitamins I feel like cow dung. I get exhausted and my stomach aches. I know for a fact if I pull the calcium out of my diet today, I will start cramping tomorrow.

I also know that in spite of all these hormones and pills, when my MS acts up, I will try anything to ease the pain. And I mean anything.

When I returned from Sweden I tried to go to the gym but I couldn't exercise the way I had been. It wasn't fatigue. I just couldn't do it; I had lost my coordination. So I threw myself into work, hoping to take my mind off the pain that way. That's when I started experimenting with Talwin, Percocet, Vicodin, Zoloft. . . . I started taking all of them just to see if I could get some kind of relief. I was calling friends who were doctors or who knew doctors who could write me a prescription . . . I was ignorant, and I was grasping at straws.

I was in search of anything that could make a difference. I went through the list of every available pharmaceutical. After Vicodin, I tried Talwin, a narcotic, and the closest thing to heroin you can legally get. It gave me a little relief, but, like Zoloft, it gave me suicidal thoughts. I found myself planning that if something went wrong in the next hour I would just kill myself. I dumped them in the toilet after taking eight or ten.

Next I tried OxyContin, an opium derivative, which is the most powerful prescription narcotic on the market. It actually worked. There's just one small problem: it's one of the most highly addictive substances around. I was popping two every four hours per the instructions, and it wasn't cooling my burning feet. What it did do was put me in never-never land. It made my thoughts race. I found myself watching the dials of my clock move and thinking about how to catch time. It shuts your intestines down. It shuts *everything* down. It's a foul drug that can do some serious damage to the liver. Finally, after I had taken eight of them, they kicked in; my pain turned off like a faucet. Unfortunately, they put me out for about nine hours. I was a zombie. I didn't realize when people were talking to me, or if I did I couldn't form a response; all I could manage was "Eeeeeeeee." So again, this may work for some—it just wasn't right for me.

The next day I woke up and was in no pain at all for three hours, which meant the drug was still in my system. It was nice to awake to no pain, but then the pain came back. So I washed down another eight pills. The third day I realized there was something wrong. I was taking too many pills and they weren't working the way I had expected. I remembered that Bret Favre, the quarterback for the Green Bay Packers, was once so addicted to a painkiller that he wound up taking handfuls of them at a time and started having seizures. Here I was, just a few days into OxyContin, and I was up to eight. What would it be the next week? That scared me. I knew people who took just one of them and became goofy, like they were inebriated. I was taking way more than that and all I was doing was putting my brain in a stupor and my pain on pause.

All the while I was experimenting with pills for the pain, of course, I was also injecting myself with the MS drug every day. The drug I'm on is an expensive drug ($40 a shot; $1,200 a month). For that kind of money you'd think it would be a marvelous drug, so wonderful it does everything but clean your teeth. Instead it can cause fever, anxiety, shortness of breath, stiffening of the chest, bumps and bruises. All the possible side effects are there in black and white on the outside of the box, and I've had every one of them. I frequently felt short of breath after taking the shot. One day I got a really ugly reaction on my left thigh, a huge bruise and a six-inch rash. A few days later I thought I was having a heart attack. At first I had some kind of side effect every other day; now I'll get a reaction every thirty or forty shots and I know it has to do with the sloppiness of the job I do.

One of the weird things about MS is that what seems to work for me doesn't necessarily work for someone else with the same symptoms. On the bright side, there are several different drugs to choose from . . . as long as you can afford them. On the down side, every one of them has adverse side effects.

And then there's the needle factor. There are no oral drugs for MS; all the drugs that have been developed are injected. At the least, dealing with the needle every single day reminds you in a very painful way that you're sick, that you're not normal.

Even worse, having to give yourself shots on a regular basis is very difficult for a lot of people. I've read that about 50 percent of the population has a fear of needles. I know for me it was a huge struggle. When I started it was ritualistic: it took me twenty minutes every day to sit there, look at the needle, and think about it, before taking the shot. It was so traumatic that for months I cried after each shot.

To add further insult, I inject HGH *twice* a day. Fortunately, that shot goes in the thigh muscle and isn't terribly painful. The ABC drug gets moved around from thigh to stomach to butt and it hurts more because it's subcutaneous; it sits under the skin and just burns intensely at the site for twenty minutes. It's almost like battery acid. In fact, a drop causes my skin to welt.

Although even today I often bleed after injecting myself, I'd say I became a master at it after about a year. But the drug companies sure don't make it easy. It drove me crazy the way they just send you these needles in the mail and expect you to deal with it. (I did have a nurse come to my office to teach me but it wasn't too successful. She was so starstruck that she was paying more attention to me than she was to telling me how to take my medication!)

With HGH I could use any size needle I wanted, so I started using the infant diabetic size. That was easy in comparison to the MS medication needle, which is prepackaged and, to me, huge. I guess there are a lot of people who can handle needles this size, but when I held the two needles side by side I said to myself, "Who the hell would choose this long, thick needle over the short, thin one?" I actually argued about this with the president of the pharmaceutical company. "Why don't you just make the needles smaller?" I asked. He insisted I was the only one who had ever complained about it.

The company wasn't about to change their needles so I started ordering smaller ones myself and transferring the medication from their syringes to my own. It's a ridiculous ordeal—pulling the plunger off the infant syringe, squirting the contents of their syringe into mine, replacing the plunger, and sticking it into my body.

But I've gotten used to the routine over the last four years. Now it's as much a part of my day as brushing my teeth, except my gums don't bleed the way my skin often does. Like most kids, mine were very uncomfortable at the thought of needles, and it freaked them out that I had to give myself shots every night. I thought it might help if I showed them how to do it, to demystify it a little bit. My girls remained somewhat squeamish, but Gooch, he got right into the spirit of it. He would happily help me find a good spot on my skin to pinch and inject, and he couldn't wait to play doctor himself. But I saw the gleam in his eye. I was thinking, "No way, man. You like it too much!" He'd say, "Please, Dad, I just want to help you."

But I'm sorry—he's still a bit young to be punching needles into his dad's butt.

I travel a lot, and I've had a problem carrying my medication with me. With the heightened security at airports these days, I'm often stopped when they see my syringes. I'm usually told they'll allow two, but not twenty, in my hand luggage. I don't get that! What difference does it make? I could do as much damage with two as I could with twenty! Which really isn't any damage at all. It's stupid because now I have to put my medication in a suitcase and wonder whether the airline is going to lose it. The whole time I'm flying I'm worrying that my bag is not going to get there. Believe me, it's happened.

But when I'm flying, or when I'm at a fancy restaurant, the one thing I no longer do is order a glass of wine. I fancy myself as rather knowledgeable about wines and I used to be a big wine drinker. No more. A doctor told me that alcohol can slow down the absorption of the drug I take. If I'm going to stick a needle in my body every day then nothing is stopping that from working.

In addition to the pills I take and the drugs I inject into my body, I'm also very mindful of my diet. I put a lot of energy into thinking through what to eat and try to adhere to it. As I have gotten older, I have cut back on the amount of red meat I eat and I try to vary the types of protein I consume from fish to chicken to supplements. I also eat four to six smaller meals a day as opposed to three large meals a day. I try to eat most of my complex carbohydrates in the morning before noon, and then eat mostly protein and anything green or dark in color the rest of the day.

Then there's the controversial issue of fillings. There's no consensus among doctors about this but I had all the amalgams in my teeth removed a year after I came back from Sweden. Pure mercury is an extremely toxic substance. It is mixed with particles of copper, silver, and tin when used as a filling in a tooth. This amalgam was thought to be stable, but mercury is not stable and it can leach into the body. I've had twenty-five doctors tell me that it doesn't really matter, but if that's true, then why has the American Academy of

Dentistry come up with a different substance to put in people's mouths from now on? They don't use mercury anymore. Maybe someone figured out that, even in small amounts, poison is poison. It leaches into your body every time you move your mouth. Doctors who have done studies on extreme mercury poisoning in South American children found all kinds of autoimmune system and neurological disorders.

Obviously, we don't yet know the whole story, but it was enough for me to remove the mercury that was in my mouth. Then I had to go through a detox period for about a month, because just taking the amalgam out of your teeth doesn't get it completely out of your system. During the removal process microscopic particles of mercury get blown up into your mouth and you swallow them and inhale them, right back into your system. So you have to detox through a whole regimen of homeopathic herbs and vitamins that I had to take on multiple occasions every day. You're supposed to do it for sixty days; I did it for thirty. I take twenty damn pills twice a day already; just taking the additional thirty or so pills was exhausting. I figured if I did half the other half will leach out eventually.

If my behavior sounds at all extreme that's because I am extreme. But remember that a lot of what I'm talking about occurred within my first year of being diagnosed. I refer to the eight months after I returned from the Karolinska Institute as my zombie period. Everyone says that the first year is the hardest because of the denial, the depression, the resistance, the distance put between you and your family and friends. That's when I let myself go the most, when I was willing to take any legally prescribed narcotic to comatose my brain and keep my pain in check. But it wasn't working. Nothing was ever enough. I was screwing up my system on a daily basis and coming back for more. I wasn't thinking clearly and I wasn't communicating well. For a TV talk show host, that wasn't a healthy situation.

When I started snowboarding, I often found myself in a lot of pain going up in the chairlift. I might have to chew six Advils, washing them down with snow. And then I tried to put my pain in a box before going down the hill.

This was a visualization technique I learned from a therapist I had seen for family counseling. It works for any kind of fear or pain. If you're afraid of the dark, you can take that darkness and put it into a box. I'd take my pain and put it in a box, tie it up, put it in the closet, shut the door, lock it in, and keep it there.

It's not easy to do. You try to pick up all the hurt but pieces will fall out, slip between your fingers; you just have to try to get as much as you can into this box. If it slides out of the box, stuff it back in. Over and over again. Once it's all in the box you close the lid.

When I do this with the fire in my feet I can make that fire go away a little. I have to fight to close the lid over and over. I usually use gaffer's tape, which works pretty well. I tie the entire box in a gaffer's tape bow, and I put the box in the closet. It's like a bad sci-fi movie—locking the terrible pain away, hoping it doesn't figure out a way to get out—but it's in the closet and it's not burning me. Then I do mental gymnastics to keep it there. This is not a once-a-day process. It's ongoing. When the pain returns, I tie it up again. It's become a part of my routine because I have mild to moderate pain twenty-four hours a day.

I've had to make some very conscious decisions to live with MS. I talk about these decisions with my kids, especially the older girls, Ashley and Maressa. I tell them about the fragility of life and how the choices we make can have far-reaching consequences. Look at me: five and ten years ago, I thought I understood everything about the choices I was making for myself, yet they could have been exacerbating a disease I didn't yet know I had. Sometimes when I'm talking about the consequences of our actions I see Ashley sit back with a look on her face that says, "Here we go again. Enough, Dad. I get it." But that doesn't stop me from talking. I have to convince them that the decision you make today can have an effect on your life years from now.

That's what I tried to tell Ashley when I put her in that boarding school in Idaho. Had she decided to cut school with her friends the day they wrapped a car around a pole, who knows if she would have made it out alive or if she could have been crippled for the rest of her life?

I love my daughter and she knows it. Everything we've been through I would not trade for the world. Sometimes my other kids have felt jealous, like they feel Ashley gets all the attention. Well, she is my firstborn child, and she's the only one with a medical issue like epilepsy. I probably cut Ashley a break that I won't cut the other children, and I'm willing to do so for the rest of her life. That doesn't mean she gets more—it means Dad understands.

In the summer of 2000 I drove to Idaho with my friend Rupert to pick her up and bring her home. As we drove along the highway on the way there we looked up ahead and noticed smoke coming from the trees below the road. A car had gone off the side of the road down into the woods and started a fire. There were already two cars stopped, so we thought we would make a quick check to see if they had called 911. I got out and yelled down the sixty-foot embankment, "Do you need some help?" Two men were just standing there, looking at this kid whose face was busted and bleeding. He had dragged himself out of the car and was lying facedown about fifteen feet away from his burning car. I yelled, "Did you guys call 911?" but they didn't move. It was like something out of the movie *Deliverance* where Jon Voight, Burt Reynolds, Ronny Cox and Ned Beatty confront these inbred backwoodsmen. Then I heard *pop pop pop* as the car's windows started exploding. The pops were so loud I thought there was a gun in the car going off. I realized we had to get out of there fast. The trees were on fire, and there's his car with a gas tank that might ignite. I climbed down the embankment and rolled the driver over.

I said, "Can you hear me?" He didn't answer; he was in shock. "Look, I'm going to touch you from head to toe and you tell me what hurts." When I got to his ankle I saw that it was broken. The other guys were still standing around in a daze, so I told them to take off their belts and I got some branches to make a splint to mobilize the kid's ankle. Then I picked him up and put him on my back and carried him up to the road. A woman driving by in a camper stopped and I asked her if she had any ice, which I used to pack his ankle. By this time a couple of other cars had stopped and someone said EMS was on the way, so Rupert and I got in our car and left.

We picked up Ashley, who was relieved to get out of what she called "prison," and drove back past the scene about an hour later. There were fire trucks and cop cars and we were waved to stop. This cop had a real angry look on his face. I thought, "I guess you really don't see a lot of black people in Idaho." The cop said someone recognized our truck as having left the scene of an accident.

"I didn't leave the scene of anything," I said. "The accident had already taken place." I took an attitude and the cop became conciliatory. He told us that the injured person was a sixteen-year-old boy on his way to football practice at his school. He had fallen asleep at the wheel and driven his car off the side of the road.

As we drove away Ashley began asking questions about what had happened and I told her about the two guys standing and looking at the kid who had crashed and how I put the kid on my back and carried him up that steep hill.

"What about your MS?" she wondered. "What were you thinking? Why didn't you let those guys carry him?"

"Because those guys weren't reacting," I said. "And at that point, all I was thinking was *MS, get out of my way!*"

I winked at my daughter as we drove away from the scene and made believe I didn't hear her murmur, "Oh, brother," as she shook her head and tried to hide the smile I saw forming on her face.

What she didn't see was that I was smiling too. My feet were hurting before I ran down to help that young man, and they were hurting after I carried him back up, but when I had him on my back, with those guys watching and not helping, my adrenaline kicked in, allowing my brain to send whatever messages it needed to send for my body to function normally. I wasn't a victim of MS in those moments. I may have been joking with Ashley when I made that play on words but for the rest of that long drive back I was thinking that MS really was just another mountain I needed to get beyond.

7

In the Eyes of the Law, I'm a Criminal

". . . to live outside the law, you must be honest."
—Bob Dylan, "Absolutely Sweet Marie"

I consider myself a responsible and caring parent who believes in discipline, respect, and good manners. So when I take a controversial stand, I do it with forethought and with seriousness. I'm not a frivolous person, and I'm nothing like Sean Penn's stoner character in *Fast Times at Ridgemont High*. If anything I am strict, orderly, abstemious, and very much in control. I like things to be in their right place.

I'm not a liberal Democrat; I have voted Republican or Independent all my life. I'm a marine who graduated from the Naval Academy and worked in sensitive, classified jobs on everything from aircraft carriers to submarines. I'm a motivational speaker who has talked to well over three million schoolchildren about making the right choices when it comes to drugs. I've done public service antidrug announcements for the White House. I'm a syndicated television talk show host who has managed to stay on the air for thirteen years. I'm a person who cares about crime, addiction, child abuse, medical care and the high cost of insurance. I'm also a person in constant pain and I don't want to become a prescription drug addict.

So I use cannabis.

Even though I use it medicinally, that still makes me, in the eyes of the law, a criminal.

I think that's wrong. There is something very archaic about the law that labels those of us who have chronic pain criminals for trying to subdue that pain and remain active and productive.

Federal law classifies drugs according to schedules, from I to V. Schedule V drugs like the cough syrup Robitussin AC and the diarrhea-stopping Lomotil are considered to have the lowest potential for abuse. Schedule IV drugs like Xanax, Valium, Ambien, and Halcion also have a low potential for abuse. Abuse of either schedule V or IV drugs "may lead to limited physical dependence or psychological dependence." Schedule III drugs, like the pure THC Marinol, anabolic steroids, barbiturates, and phenobarbital have a "*moderate*" potential for abuse. Schedule II—amphetamines, cocaine, codeine, methadone, morphine, and opium—have a high potential for abuse, which may lead to "*severe* psychological or physical dependence." The United States allows some medicinal use of Schedule II drugs, but with heavy restrictions. Then there is Schedule I. These drugs are banned, considered unsafe to use even under medical supervision, with a high potential for abuse. PCP, LSD, heroin and Quaaludes are classified Schedule I. And so is marijuana.

This has got to change.

Would I legalize heroin in America? No.

Would I legalize Ecstasy? No.

Would I encourage children under voting age to use any kind of drug? Absolutely not.

Are there certain drugs I would legalize for medicinal purposes, which would then generate revenue for this country to deal with addiction? Yes! I think it's feasible, and I think it would be smart.

This is something the leaders of this country don't want to hear. They will talk about how they are against drugs and in favor of protecting our children, yet they will allow the highly addictive substance called alcohol to pervade every aspect of a child's life. Every time our children turn on the television to watch a sporting event they see beer commercials. Picnics, celebrations, BBQs, ballparks—

we're teaching them that wherever there is "fun" and "good times" there's alcohol. In magazines, on radio and television, we are inundated ten times an hour by ads for drugs: if you don't feel great take an antidepressant or an ibuprofen or an over-the-counter medicine that might damage your liver. It's shoved down our throats and then we wonder why this nation has an addiction problem. But we won't talk about that.

We don't need any more studies to know the effects of too much alcohol in our systems. We don't need further tests showing that taking more than three aspirin at a time can cause serious damage to your stomach, and taking a handful is a suicide attempt. And by now we really don't need to test marijuana to know that it can get you high.

Well, we also know it relieves pain, and it isn't addictive. Anyone who says otherwise is ignorant.

Way back in 1938, New York mayor Fiorello La Guardia appointed a committee to study marijuana. The committee consisted of the commissioners of Corrections, Health, and Hospitals, the director of the Division of Psychiatry of the Department of Hospitals, two pharmacologists, two internists, and three psychiatrists. It took them six years to present their findings: marijuana didn't cause aggressive or antisocial behavior; it wasn't sexually overstimulating; it didn't change personalities; it didn't cause major crimes. All those myths that had created the passage of the Marijuana Tax Act of 1937 were dispelled, but the Federal Bureau of Narcotics was not going to take these findings to heart. Even though La Guardia remained New York's mayor until 1945, the study was largely ignored.

Forty-three years later, in 1988, the Drug Enforcement Administration's administrative law judge, Francis L. Young, presided over public hearings that lasted two years to consider reclassifying marijuana from Schedule I to Schedule II. Judge Young concluded that marijuana's classification should be changed, saying, "Marijuana, in its natural form, is one of the safest therapeutically active substances known to man. . . . One must reasonably conclude that there is accepted safety for use of marijuana under medical supervision. To conclude otherwise, on the record, would be unreasonable, arbitrary,

and capricious." Yet the DEA ignored Young's conclusions and refused to reclassify marijuana.

In 1999, the Institute of Medicine, a branch of the National
Academy of Sciences, released a two-year study of the marijuana
plant identifying more than sixty kinds of cannabinoids and their
specific actions on the brain and the body. They recommended that
the government pay for research that would speed up the development of more cannabinoid drugs. This was the study that showed
marijuana was effective in combating the muscle spasms associated
with MS.

That same year, the Ninth U.S. Circuit Court of Appeals said the
government has yet to identify any interest it may have in blocking
the distribution of marijuana to those with medical need. It found
that legal alternatives to marijuana don't work or cause intolerable
side effects.

And yet, in 2002, a DEA spokesman reacting to the passing of
California's Proposition 215 to allow patients to use marijuana to
alleviate pain, nausea, and lack of appetite said: "There is no such
thing as medical marijuana. We are Americans first, Californians
second."

Americans first? What does that mean? Am I un-American because
I would rather use pot than OxyContin, natural weed rather than
synthetic Marinol? How hypocritical can these government officials get?

I've been to congressional events and dinners where all the con-
gressmen are sitting around with drinks in their hands pontificating
about how smoking a joint is a crime and a sin. It's ridiculous. Like
other controversial issues, there are people who will never back
down on marijuana. Yet these same people think nothing of attending a rally to fight against it with beers in their hands. God knows
we promote every other drug under the sun, making sure that no
matter what your problem is you take something for it—as long as
whatever you take is going to produce the greatest profit margin for
the pharmaceutical companies, who contribute heavily to both political parties. It's no secret that these companies stand to lose billions
of dollars annually if marijuana were legal in the United States and

cultivated and sold by the government. Or simply grown in one's garden next to the rosebush and the cacti.

To convince the federal government of the benefits of marijuana as medicine requires clinical trials; but the government insists that clinical trials are unwarranted because no solid evidence exists of pot's medical value. Hello? Has anybody ever heard of catch-22? The government controls the marijuana that they would accept for testing, but they won't grant approval for any tests. Scientists can obtain pot only from the National Institute of Drug Abuse, which gets it from a government-approved farm in Mississippi. NIDA insists that researchers who apply for the plant must have their studies approved by the National Institutes of Health. The National Institutes of Health checks with the Drug Enforcement Agency, which insists that no American independent research or federal health program should be allowed to investigate natural cannabis derivatives for medicine. They just make you go around in circles until finally you stop trying. Scientists like Paul Consroe, a professor at the University of Arizona Health Sciences Center, feel frustrated by the Kafkaesque bureaucratic maze the government has created to keep acceptable studies of marijuana from being done or, if done, from being publicized. "Marijuana has been studied to death," Consroe says. "It's not a question of science; it's a political drug."

Why all the fear surrounding marijuana? Is it because youth in the sixties turned marijuana into a fun drug and smoked it in defiance of their parents' wishes? Is it because there's a perception that medicinal use of marijuana will eventually lead to its legalization?

Look, it doesn't have to be legalized, just decriminalized. There are millions of pot smokers who defy the law every day of the year in America. In six years the number of marijuana arrests increased from 481,098 in 1994 to 734,500 in 2000. That's three-quarters of a million people a year being jailed for using a naturally grown weed! As for the medical use of marijuana, all we want is for seriously ill people to be allowed to seek physician-recommended relief from their illness and not be arrested for their efforts.

In our society today, with Big Brother encroaching more and

more on our privacy and our liberties in the name of homeland security, it is probably foolhardy to take a stand, but sometimes foolhardiness is a catalyst for social change. Lots of folks thought the guys who sat in a room to come up with the Declaration of Independence were foolhardy too; but they saw that change was necessary. I don't know if I'd call them foolhardy, but some of them were definitely putting weed in their pipes when they weren't going to their snuffboxes. It was even recently reported that pot residue was found in one of Benjamin Franklin's pipes!

Most of the founding fathers grew or smoked pot. Thomas Jefferson preferred growing hemp over tobacco—he believed that hemp was more important to the wealth and protection of the country, because hemp had so many uses: as a natural fiber, as a yarn for rope, for paper, as an oil for cooking, as a fuel, as a way to aerate soil and control erosion, as medicine, as a source of protein, and as a way to stimulate creativity. The sails that helped carry Christopher Columbus and his crew across the Atlantic were made of hemp. The first two drafts of the Declaration of Independence were written on hemp. Native Americans used it in ceremonies along with peyote because they believed it opened your mind and freed your ingenuity. There are reports of marijuana being used as a medicine that go much further back—back to China in 4000 B.C., as well as to India, the Middle East, Southeast Asia, South Africa, and South America, all before the birth of Christ. It was used to lower fever, cure malaria, ease constipation, lessen rheumatic pains; to induce sleep, for dysentery, to stimulate appetite, improve digestion, reduce headaches, and as an analgesic during surgery. Hemp oil was used to treat coughs, venereal disease, and urinary incontinence. In 1621 a European clergyman named Robert Burton wrote *The Anatomy of Melancholy*, in which he described using it as a treatment for depression. In the last half of the nineteenth century there were over a hundred papers published in medical literature recommending it. According to one of President Kennedy's mistresses, Judith Exner, JFK smoked marijuana in the White House, and we know today how much pain he was in.

It really is a miracle plant. Like the peanut, its uses are almost innumerable. The jeans I wear are made from hemp. So are some of my shirts. Certain plastics are hardened with hemp fibers. It can be used to make paint, varnishes, soap and linoleum. The seeds can feed birds and the residue, livestock. It can make dioxin-free white paper to use as toilet paper, newspaper, stationery, book paper, paper towels, Dixie cups, and milk cartons. Cannabis seeds are the richest source of essential fatty oils that support the immune system and guard against viral attacks. Hemp seed oil can be used as an alternative fuel. It's crazy that to end our dependence on Middle Eastern oil we're not looking at those kinds of viable options.

I'm not making any of this up—there are 389 carefully researched books dealing with marijuana available at Amazon.com; 331 at BarnesandNoble.com. None of them are in the fiction section. There is a wealth of information at Marijuana.com. Check it out yourself.

Laws prohibiting alcohol were passed in the 1920s and against marijuana in the 1930s. But the laws prohibiting the use of alcohol were repealed, and now as you're reading these words a drunk driver will kill himself and/or someone else; some inebriated tough guy will pull a knife on some other poor bastard in a bar; a jerk in an alcoholic stupor will assault a young woman on a college campus or a city street. But that's just the cost of doing business, and in America, liquor is big business. Marijuana, on the other hand, is still illegal, and one must wonder why. There's no big business lobbying for it, just some hundreds of thousands of people suffering from diseases, people in pain looking for relief, and millions of young people looking to get high so they can get into their favorite music at concerts and parties, mellowing and chilling and acting the exact opposite of those drunken boors whose behavior is not just offensive but dangerous.

I can go to my local supermarket or liquor store, buy myself a bottle of tequila, whiskey, scotch, or gin and guzzle myself into the gutter. Nobody can do anything about it. Or I can take a pinch of kef, put it in a tiny glass bowl the size of my small fingernail and smoke it and be liable to arrest, trial, legal expenses, and jail time.

We claim to be a compassionate nation and care about those in need. We have bills written to protect patients from being ripped off, overcharged, and improperly diagnosed (though that doesn't keep these things from happening), but here is something that can, without question, help patients who are in pain or depressed, that can prevent us from sitting at home all night suffering silently by ourselves, and all we are asking is to be allowed to use it.

The rules and regulations that make it almost impossible to effectively research this substance via federally sanctioned testing must be changed. They date back to 1937, after Henry J. Anslinger, the director of the Federal Bureau of Narcotics (which would evolve into the DEA) testified before Congress: "Marijuana is the most violence-causing drug in the history of mankind." What a crock! Anslinger was to pot what Senator Joe McCarthy was to Communism. They both created fear by accentuating the negative, negating the factual, and by the sheer force of their personalities pushed forward policies that have not served this country well. Anslinger's crusade against marijuana nearly seventy years ago is one of the last bastions of the old blue laws that in some states prohibit oral sex or mixed marriages.

Most of the misinformation on marijuana, and most of the reasons people get so upset about it, are based on a mentality that existed prior to television, computers, cell phones, space shuttles and about 90 percent of everything we take for granted today. It's time to update that information.

There's a moment in Nikos Kazantzakis's book *Zorba the Greek* when Zorba asks his young educated boss, "Why do the young die?" And his boss answers that he doesn't know. Exasperated, Zorba challenges him: "What's the use of all your damn books? If they can't answer that, what the hell *do* they tell you?"

"They tell me," his boss replies, "of the agony of men who can't answer questions like yours."

It's a clever response, but not a satisfactory answer. The young shouldn't die, but they do. And those who don't die from war or accident or natural disasters mostly die from illness. They die from AIDS, from leukemia, from suicidal depression, from any number of things. And if they make it past their youth, then they die in their prime, or in middle age. And before they die they suffer.

If Zorba was transplanted to today he might ask a politician, "Why do the sick have to suffer?" And after getting some typical politician's nonanswer he might say, "What's the use of all the damn studies if they're suppressed or ignored?"

If the politician stays true to the party line his answer might be, "Because the law says it doesn't help, even if those who use it claim it does. And the law supersedes right or wrong. It supersedes ethics, morality, compassion, and understanding."

To which I say, like the rebellious mutants in *The Island of Dr. Moreau*, "Law no more!"

Those who suffer from any number of diseases who have received relief from their symptoms after smoking or ingesting marijuana have three choices: to do nothing and live with their pain; to take the prescribed drugs that are costly, have serious side effects, and may cause addiction; or ingest or smoke a little pot. The naysayers, our lawmakers, want to deny us the least harmful and least expensive choice and prefer we become a nation of addicts instead. Because the pharmaceutical companies and the tobacco companies and the liquor companies aren't going to get rich if people stop paying for their products and instead throw some seeds into a planter or in their backyards and harvest that. And that's, really, what it comes down to. Deep Throat told Woodward and Bernstein to "follow the money" to uncover the Watergate scandal. That's the way it has always been. That's why the federal government hasn't given in to the will of the people in the thirty-five states that have ratified laws surrounding medicinal marijuana. The lobbyists are just too strong, the politicians are just too weak, and no president has yet been brave enough to take a moral and compassionate stand.

I believe President Bush is one of the more centered presidents we've ever had. I don't really think he's the Republican people think he is, and he's not as soft as some think he is. He's a guy riding both parties who has alienated some of his own party as well as some Democrats. If he can navigate the waters he's in to at least change the tide on some domestic issues, he might end up leaving a surprising legacy. I believe he's very forward thinking. I believe if anyone were to legalize marijuana for medicinal purposes it might be him. He also understands the economic ramifications of marijuana. He just needs to be pushed in the right direction to get that done.

I know that his administration is against it, but if I had a chance to sit with him in the Oval Office I would tell him this:

"I'm coming to you, Mr. President, to ask for your compassion. You have two daughters—if one of them was hurting, would you, as president of the United States, stand by and allow your child to suffer? Your brother, the governor of Florida, has a child who was hurting and he decided to do what was necessary to help her before he allowed the law to step in. He put his daughter, your niece, in rehabilitation centers multiple times because he was compassionate enough to understand she didn't need to go to jail—she needed help.

"People who have MS don't need to go to jail—we need help. There are legal drugs that work for some people, but for people like myself who suffer from extreme pain and tremors that disrupt our sleep, when these drugs don't work, this is my only option. Why does the government feel the need to eradicate this plant from the face of the earth when it has been doing so much good for so many thousands of years? The law that says marijuana is a Schedule I drug and has no proven medicinal value is unsupported by scientific data.

"Mr. President, the most compassionate thing you can do is make me stop believing in a false panacea. Help me stop thinking that something that's really harmful to me, such as prescribed addictive drugs that often cause serious side effects, is helpful. Why don't you launch an initiative to truly research the viability of cannabis as a drug? Commission a panel that can study it independently."

So far the only time the government has been willing to test marijuana is when they have a specific agenda, which is to keep it from being used. When their own test results prove otherwise, they ignore the tests.

When drug companies submit their studies of high-priced painkillers, they aren't met with an attitude that says, "Ha! These drugs will never be approved." But bring up marijuana, which has only been around for six thousand years, and it's like the thought police come out of the closet and just shut down any rationality.

In Canada, up in Manitoba, they have this place called the Rock, where the government grows marijuana. They're working a lot with MS sufferers because they have a large cluster of them in Manitoba and Winnipeg. The Netherlands permits pharmacies to dispense marijuana to people with cancer, AIDS, MS and Tourette's syndrome to treat pain, nausea, loss of appetite, to alleviate spasm pains and reduce tics. Great Britain also decriminalized pot for medicinal purposes based on an exhaustive study. You can get a prescription there. There is scientific data out there on marijuana in Canada, Israel, the Netherlands and England. Why not in the United States?

Look at the white willow tree. It's a difficult tree that does a lot of damage in the forest; it's hard to grow other plants near it. There was probably a time in history when people would have liked to get rid of the tree. Then we found out that it had medicinal value, that chewing the bark relieved pain. Of course we're not into bark-chewing these days, so what did we do? We took that tree apart and figured out a way to synthesize the active ingredient and create a tablet—aspirin—that was more palatable than chewing on bark. We've used marijuana at least as long as we have the willow tree or any of the other thousands of plants found in the forest that have medicinal value. Why don't we figure out a way to process it and make it like an aspirin? If investigated and studied honestly there will be irrefutable evidence that it is a positive, powerful drug.

One of the biggest fallacies is that marijuana will lead to harder drugs. That's one of the reasons why our endless war against drugs has failed: because the public is being lied to. Marijuana is *not* going to make you run out and become a heroin addict. It's *not* going to destroy your brain cells. It *doesn't* impair memory or cognition. It *doesn't* interfere with our sex hormones. It *doesn't* impair our immune systems. It is *not* highly addictive. It *isn't* more damaging to the lungs than tobacco. It *does* have medicinal value.

Tens of thousands of patients across America are using medicinal marijuana even though the federal penalty is up to one year in prison for possessing a single joint, and up to five years for a plant. In Humboldt County, California, recently, Christopher Krohn, the mayor of

Santa Cruz, along with several city council members and two former mayors, witnessed a medical marijuana giveaway on the steps of City Hall. "This is not an attempt to embarrass the DEA," he said, "but rather a compassionate gathering in support of sick people who need their medicine." We're going to see more and more civil disobedience as more and more patients rebel against the high cost of the drugs they're prescribed and the terrible side effects so many of them have. At the end of the day we will have ended up spending, who knows, a half a trillion dollars on the war with Iraq, and we could have spent less than .01 percent of that to research marijuana. For about 10 percent we could probably find cures for cancer, AIDS, and MS.

Dr. Lester Grinspoon, an associate professor of psychiatry at Harvard Medical School, has said, "This country has devoted millions of dollars, mainly through NIDA, to establish the toxicity of marijuana. They've come up with a goose egg." The reason, of course, is that marijuana is nontoxic. No one has ever OD'd from just smoking pot. To do that, you'd have to smoke the equivalent of half a million joints in a row—and you'd probably die from emphysema before you died from the active ingredient in pot.

Marijuana has some negatives, without a doubt—it can affect your lungs if you smoke it in heavy doses, and certain genetically altered pot has a higher concentration of THC, which makes it stronger—but would I really be better off using morphine instead to relieve my pain? My doctor tells me I could become addicted. He warned that I'd have to bear the brunt of about fifty other detrimental side effects to avoid pain. Same thing with Percocet and a number of other Schedule II drugs that are out there.

A 1991 Harvard study of oncologists found that 44 percent of the cancer specialists recommended patients break the law to obtain the marijuana they medically required. I agree with Dr. Grinspoon, who pointed out that "the government's position against clinical trials is immoral, illegal, and certainly unscientific."

We need to stop screwing around and do the research that will settle this question. If the research comes back and says unequivocally there is no efficacy to marijuana for any illness then I will be the first person to stand up and say I was wrong; but I doubt that's going to happen.

In spite of the fact that our government has made federally sanctioned testing so difficult, we have learned more about the chemistry of marijuana during the past ten years perhaps than in the previous six thousand years combined.

In the early 1990s, the discovery of receptors in the brain for molecules of the cannabinoids in marijuana triggered massive scientific interest in the health effects of marijuana. Scientists have found an interrelationship between the cannabinoid receptors and the opium receptors in the brain. We know that both opium and marijuana have the ability to inhibit the perception of pain. We know that opium and marijuana are both natural products. We know that morphine, an opium derivative that is highly addictive, is prescribed for its pain-blunting properties. Yet marijuana, which is not addictive, is illegal. We know that morphine causes gastrointestinal side effects while marijuana has a positive impact on appetite. So why does the government encourage one natural plant product for alleviating pain and ban the other?

If marijuana was in the same Schedule II category as morphine, then it could be mixed with the more addictive opiate to increase morphine's biological activity and lessen its potential for addiction. Better to combine marijuana with morphine than to prescribe morphine alone. And better still, forget the morphine and use marijuana alone to lessen and more probably avoid the side effects and addiction altogether.

If I were president I would immediately commission a definitive study on the use of marijuana in all its derivations and forms. Just like they had to do when aspirin first came around—it was an alternative medicine when it was first marketed. We should take the plant apart, identify the active ingredients that cause the euphoria and the pain relief, and then without attempting to synthesize it, actually collect it like you do other plants that we use.

I would set up viable tests at several universities and provide government funds for independent, not government, studies. While that is going on I would collate all the known side effects—not from some agency clones down in Washington, D.C., but from independent sources. As with tobacco, smoking marijuana could be bad for the lungs. So how much can you safely smoke in a week? I think that could be figured out easily. Then I'd come up with what they do for all drugs: a risk assessment. So if I'm going to work at lessening my pain but I know that in taking this tablet I stand the chance of developing something down the road, it's my option. If I understand it and if I still choose to do it then Uncle Sam should utilize the resources that we have in place to grow and cultivate this plant in the cleanest form they can, which is hydroponically, as in Canada.

Then I would prescribe it medicinally.

Right now I would not make it legal but I would decriminalize possession of small amounts for medicinal purposes. Someone who has five thousand cases of scotch in their house that they brought across the Canadian border is going to get busted and go to jail for illegally distributing alcohol. Same should be true with weed.

I would set up government stations to package and sell it because there's going to be a large profit margin. The profits could fund rehabilitation of those addicted to other drugs. That would lessen the burden on the U.S. legal system, because marijuana is not the drug of choice when it comes to robbing liquor stores or holding up old ladies. I have never heard a newscast reporting, "John Smith was high on marijuana when he robbed this store—or when he assaulted this person. . . ." It doesn't happen. High on crack or PCP, yes. Marijuana doesn't make you violent; it relaxes you. That's why it's been called "mellow yellow." So the chances of seeing crime and aberrant behavior go up are very slim, especially if Uncle Sam is the one controlling it.

So if I were president I would (1) test, (2) grow, (3) distribute it for medicinal purposes with a prescription, (4) decriminalize small quantities. I would put the sale and distribution of it in the same category as alcohol to keep it away from minors. And (5) I would change its status from Schedule I to Schedule IV or V. It would remain a prescription medicine and the insurance companies would have to kick in a subsidy, so those patients who couldn't otherwise afford it could benefit from it.

I've asked doctors about using medical marijuana and off the record they tell me if it works to alleviate my pain and tremors to go ahead and use it. Because of this almost neo-Nazi attitude toward marijuana and anyone who speaks out about it, most doctors are scared even to say anything because of possible repercussions from their boards of health and from politicians.

However, in the last five years doctors have finally begun to understand that they need to allow patients, especially the chronically ill, to be more responsible for handling their pain. That's the reason why after surgery most hospitals put patients on a pump by which they can administer their own pain relief. Thank God we're starting to become a little more compassionate as a society. There was a time when the doctors decreed how much you would get and when, leaving patients to suffer needlessly. Now, by pressing a button, patients can get as much pain relief as they want, when they want it. And surprise: studies show they use less medication, not more, when it's in their control.

I'm not a hospital patient but there should be a way for me to manage my own pain based on what works for me. It would be really hard for me to be a heroin addict; I don't have the correct receptor for it. Anything that's opium-based doesn't do that much for me, other than cause constipation. Percocet helps other people but all it does for me is keep me from going to the bathroom for a month.

Smoking pot should not be looked at as degenerate. I know someone with MS who had never smoked marijuana in his life. He'd been taking Tylenol with codeine for a year to no avail, and his doctor told him to increase the number he was taking. Instead he was given some liquid cannabis to squeeze through a dropper on his food and it's helped him where the narcotics did not. He now swears by it.

I have spasms in my sleep that make me shake and kick. It'll last for about five minutes, then I'll go into a cramp and the pain of the cramp is what wakes me up. I tried two antitremor drugs but I didn't like them. Marijuana, however, will stop these tremors immediately.

I don't use it when my pain has subsided. And I prefer eating it to smoking. When they say it's time to set the record straight, the record should show that it doesn't have to only be smoked; it can be ingested or inhaled using the kind of inhalator asthma patients use. You filter out some of the harmful chemicals by using a vaporizer, passing it through water before it goes into your system. Or you extract the compounds in the pot that help reduce the pain and make it into pastes, jellies and seasonings for food. It has fewer carcinogens in it than most of what we grow on farms to sell to the public.

The evidence seems to show that the positives far outweigh the negatives when it comes to allowing the medicinal use of marijuana. When you factor in that it's readily available, easy to use, and relatively inexpensive compared to the cost of equivalent prescription drugs (and there really aren't any quite equivalent!), one can only raise a fist in frustration and a voice in anger that it's still illegal.

Even before I was diagnosed with MS I believed in the medicinal use of marijuana. As you can see, since being diagnosed I haven't changed my mind.

In the two decades since Nancy Reagan's "Just Say No" campaign we have spent 100 billion taxpayer dollars on the war on drugs. In 1999 alone the government spent $7.7 billion to enforce marijuana laws. Since 1965 an estimated 10 million people have been arrested for using marijuana. Nearly 1.5 million were incarcerated in just two years, 2000 and 2001. And yet the number of people in the United States who smoke marijuana increased, not decreased, to a conservative estimate of over 30 million people. They're not saying no, because they know when they're being lied to. What we're doing, in effect, is spending an inordinate amount of money to help disease the nation. Because once you put these people in prison you make them bitter. Pot users who get sentenced to five years in jail may get out in nine months, but they're going to have a federal record, they're not going to be able to get a job so easily, they'll have to lie on many kinds of job applications and they thus become a part of America's contamination.

We don't need to be locking people up for five to sixty years for a bag of marijuana. We had a girl who was an incest survivor on our show. She had been raped for eight years by her father and they gave him thirteen months in prison. Something is wrong here!

Congress made a mistake in 1970 when it passed the Comprehensive Drug Abuse Prevention and Control Act, which grouped cannabis with PCP, LSD, and heroin and classified it as having no medical use with a high potential for abuse. Mistakes get made. We never should have allowed mercury to be put in our bodies. We never should have allowed the drug thalidomide, which caused babies to be born without limbs, to be given to pregnant women. And we never should have incarcerated so many of our best and brightest for smoking a joint, or for growing it for medicinal purposes. We have entered the twenty-first century. The time has come to admit to our mistakes and move forward, not backward.

8

I Saw a Cloud Coming up the Hudson

In the last thirteen years, I've done twenty-six hundred television shows and not one of them dealt with the subject of medical marijuana. I've read a lot about it, but until working on this book I hadn't put it all together. Before this I didn't feel I could do a responsible show about it and I wouldn't be able to take the heat if I tried. Most people who have discussed the subject have been looked upon as charlatans or cranks, because the government has controlled the media in the way it looks at marijuana. I didn't want to jump into that fray completely unarmed and without the nation being ready to hear it. Now, this nation is ready. We have a governor in California, Mr. Schwarzenegger, who believes strongly in medicinal marijuana. We have thirty-five states that have already passed some sort of legislation to lessen the penalties for using it. And we've just had the Supreme Court saying the administration was wrong in attempting to prosecute doctors who consider compassionate care their number-one priority.

I am now prepared to do whatever it takes to make people understand that being for medicinal marijuana is being for compassionate care. I'm ready to do shows about the subject with both advocates and naysayers. I'd want to balance any show with those who believe it's a worthy cause and those who feel it's a criminal violation of our laws and ethics. Let them bring their facts and data.

I brought mine to high schools around the country before I became a talk show host. While still a naval officer, I talked about negative youth trends: dropping out, drugging out and sexing out. Peer pressuring out. This was back in early 1988, when America was at the height of the crack epidemic. I was in a navy uniform talking to kids about staying away from drugs and aberrant sexual behavior. I spoke about teenage pregnancy and being tricked into doing things you shouldn't be doing. I was speaking directly and frankly and the kids responded to what I had to say. They screamed and cheered, and it soon became a media event. The local news would cover these talks. Some of them were simulcast to fifty schools at one time. I was being interviewed by reporters from Iowa to Seattle, New York to Arkansas after each talk. In June 1988, I was featured on the *NBC Nightly News*. The next day I was talking to Jane Pauley on the *Today* show. It made me realize that we were a nation starving for leadership when it came to what to do with and for our children. I resigned my naval commission after seventeen years in the service and decided to do this full-time. People told me I was crazy, but by then I had spoken to 100,000 kids in thirty different schools. What crossed my mind was that these kids in ten years would be in their mid to late twenties and voting. I wasn't thinking about becoming a talk show host. I was thinking about running for president.

For the next three years I continued speaking to students. In 1990 I was approached by a Gannett TV station in Florida to do a simulcast. That show won them a Best of Gannett award for the year. I was then asked to do similar shows for other Gannett stations. I did a number of them, none of which paid me. Then a woman who worked for a TV station in Denver came to me and asked if I'd do a show about the race problem they were having. I did it as a prime-time public service special and afterward people complimented me for being a great host on that show. Host? I never thought of myself as a host, but that's what I was. I wound up winning an Emmy as Best Talk Show Host for that show. And that's when I started thinking of developing a talk show.

On December 23, 1990, I met with Freddie Fields, who had executive produced *Glory* with Denzel Washington. I had done an introduction to that film for schools and that led to my meeting Fields. I showed him a poorly shot pilot I had thrown together and by January 15 I took my first meeting with Paramount. Two weeks later there was a bidding war among five syndicators for *The Montel Williams Show*. I was about to become the first African-American man to have his own daytime talk show. On April 21, 1991, I signed a contract and was on the air May 8.

The first year I did the show, it was at CBS Television City in L.A. I was up against and compared to Oprah, Phil Donahue, and Sally Jessy Raphael right from the start, though I wasn't yet a national show. Having been a motivational speaker trying to make a difference, I wanted my show to make a difference. My first edict to my producers was: we're going to do a show that doesn't belabor what happened, we're going to try to figure out *why* things happen and come up with solutions. That's what differentiated my show from the beginning, and that's also what my life is about. I'm not going to sit and cry about MS; I'm trying to figure out why there is MS and then how to cure it.

Over these thirteen years we've averaged eight to ten guests per show. That's 21,000 people sitting within arm's reach of me. The reason I've been able to understand pain and suffering is that I can read people; I can look someone in the eye and within the first three minutes tell whether that person is full of it or is someone of substance. I've had people come on my show to talk about something silly or humorous and said to them: "This isn't fun for you, is it?" I saw that one woman had marks on the back of her neck and I asked if her husband beat her. Her husband was sitting in the front row, but that show took on an entirely different meaning. Within five minutes I had that woman taken from our set to a battered women's shelter; her husband was held back by our security guards. A hundred times on my show I've looked into the eyes of a guest who came to talk about something else and asked: Were you molested when you were younger? They were, and they came to tell me that, but they used another premise to get there.

I have talked on the air to people like Mary Vincent, who at age fifteen in 1978 had run away from home. She got picked up on a highway in California by one of the most notorious serial killers in our history—nobody knows how many people he killed. He raped and brutalized her, and then took a dull ax and chopped off her arms, leaving her on the side of the road to die. I had her on the show in the early nineties and gave her the first opportunity to tell her story to a national audience. We got 50,000 phone calls in response to that show. In spite of what had happened to her, she wasn't a quitter. Through her pain, she succeeded. She came on the show a second time and brought me a picture she'd drawn with her toes—it's the best picture of me ever done. It looks like a photograph. I drew incredible strength out of that.

Another woman we had on, Barb Tarbox, was a successful Canadian model. Her mother died of lung cancer, and nineteen years later she was diagnosed with it. She realized it was a struggle she was going to lose and started speaking throughout Canada about the dangers of cigarettes. She went through chemo and radiation and went to schools, taking off her wig, to show people a balding, frail woman up until two weeks before her death. She used the pain of her own illness to educate people, to help prevent young people from going through what she was going through. This happened after my diagnosis and gave me strength to make sure I work as hard as I can to find a cure for MS.

This is the point of our show: not to rehash what happened but to figure out why things happen and to try and come up with solutions. That's why we came up with the After Care program. No show other than news shows ever had a staff psychologist. Ours runs our After Care program, which was established because one day on the show I said to a young girl suffering from an eating disorder, "I will get you help." And the next week came that woman who was being abused by her husband and I said the same thing to her. We've put more than four hundred people through our After Care program—bringing them to treatment programs dealing with drug abuse, reconstructive plastic surgery, eating disorders, interventions in spousal abuse.

There are usually two hundred people at any taping of my show and I'll sometimes ask those who are suffering from any illness or disease to raise their hands. "Who's just had bypass surgery? Who has a loaner heart? Who's just come from chemotherapy? Who has cancer?" Usually fifteen hands go up. All of these people look fine. And yet we equate illness with weakness. If you're ill you must look ill. If you don't look ill you can't be ill. But you don't have to see illness to know it's there. It's there.

Some of the shows that have touched me the most are the ones I've done with people who have MS but don't look ill. On October 25, 1999, I did the first of three shows devoted to that subject. I had four young women who let my viewers know how difficult it often is to be diagnosed with this disease and how they've managed to survive their illness. Debi told how her symptoms started when her foot fell asleep and by the end of the night she was numb all the way up to her hip. She began bumping into walls and falling down, feeling a type of vertigo where everything was constantly spinning "like an out-of-control merry-go-round." That lasted for two months. She had to be retaught how to talk, how to brush her teeth, how to walk. Her symptoms got progressively worse and she had to undergo chemotherapy for two years. She became understandably negative and depressed. And yet she came on to say that none of this stopped her from entering modeling school and participating in the Miss Massachusetts USA beauty pageant.

Lindsey started getting sick at the age of eleven but wasn't diagnosed until she turned fifteen, when she lost feeling in her left leg, had double vision and slurred speech. "I sounded like I was drunk when I really wasn't," she told us. She had problems with incontinence. Eleven doctors failed to see that she had MS until she was given an MRI and then a spinal tap.

Shawna had a brain tumor when she was seventeen and went through radiation that eradicated the cancer. But then she became temporarily paralyzed on one side. Her doctors said it was radiation relapse. She found a new neurologist who told her she had MS.

Kate was fifteen when she came on the show. She had been diagnosed with MS when she was nine. "One day after school I had a seizure for about six hours and ended up in a coma for five days," she said. She came out of that coma but could no longer attend school and had to be homeschooled.

The entertainer Lola Falana also came on that first show to talk about her battle with MS. "The first time something went wrong was in 1982," she said. "I started staggering all over the place, performing on stage like a drunken person." Five years later her left side became paralyzed. "I was half blind, half deaf, half mute. I was slurring my talk and I was dribbling out of the corner of my mouth. My hand was like a claw." She went to a neurologist who gave her an MRI and a spinal tap and told her, "There's nothing in the world that can help you." That's when she heard a voice in her head saying, "Do not let them touch you." For Lola, it was the voice of God. Today she rests for twelve hours a day and has been fine since hearing that voice.

On April 25, 2000, we did a second MS show. This time Nancy Davis came on to tell her story, how she was diagnosed at thirty-three and was convinced her life was over. "I was a young mom; I had three children. I started losing the feeling in my fingertips in my right hand, in my whole hand, in my left hand. Then I lost the feeling in my stomach, and then I lost my eyesight." But she didn't listen to the doctor who told her there was nothing to be done. She got a second opinion. And then a third opinion. And a fourth opinion. "They all confirmed I had MS, but they gave me different prognoses. And not all doctors will tell you the same thing. You cannot let a doctor play God for you. You need to be proactive and you need to ask the questions." Nancy became so proactive that she started the Center Without Walls and the annual Race to Erase MS fund-raiser.

Andrea was also a young mom when she felt "a bolt of lightning that would shoot from the top of my head all the way into my toes" every time she bent over. She couldn't feel her legs and lost the hearing in her left ear, as well as any sensation in her hands. "I can't feel if my kids' hair feels soft or it's like hay."

Then we had on Leah, eighteen, who had been diagnosed with an acute form of MS at sixteen. She lost her ability to write, she would shake, and the kids at her school shied away from her because there were rumors that it was contagious.

Our third MS show was on April 25, 2001, where a woman named Jenna described her husband Dan's progressive battle with the disease. "Dan started getting sick a little after we were married. He started losing hearing in his left ear and going numb on the left side of his body. Dan no longer can walk without assistance. He no longer can make himself his meals. He no longer can shave. He can't tie his shoes anymore."

Another man, Mark, wasn't so incapacitated. He was a trial lawyer whose biggest MS symptom was fatigue. The stress of his job and his MS affected his performance. "Imagine paying a lawyer a lot of money and all of a sudden the lawyer yawns. It's terrible."

Race car driver Kelly Sutton lost all feeling on her right side and was diagnosed with MS at sixteen, but that didn't stop her from racing. Her crew constructed a suit that runs cool air to her helmet when she's driving. "My dream came true this year," she told us proudly. "I raced Daytona and I came across that checkered flag; it was very emotional."

Then we had a long-distance runner, Susan, whose initial symptoms were loss of vision and then a tingling in her hands and feet. When she ran her first marathon her legs went out from under her. But she never gave up. She ran a few five- and ten-kilometer mini-marathons, and then she completed the Chicago Marathon, finishing the 26.2 miles in four hours and fifty-eight minutes.

What I was attempting to do with these shows was demonstrate the different faces of MS. None of these people seemed to suffer from the same symptoms, yet all of them had been diagnosed as having MS. I also brought on different doctors—Dr. Stephen Hauser, Dr. Allen Counter, Dr. Howard Weiner—to explain where they thought MS was and where it was going. All of them seemed encouraged by the advances in drugs and blood tests, new techniques with MRIs, and the new genome project; they felt we were learning more and more about the disease. Dr. Hauser went so far as to say: "For the first time in history, we have the tools that we need to get to the bottom of this disease, to develop treatments that get rid of all of the symptoms and to develop preventions that can protect people from having this disease before it begins."

I sure hope he is right.

Has my being diagnosed changed the way I do my show? It's made me a better host because it's made me a better person. Before, I could get angry about a lot of things for a long period of time. Now, I've learned to use that anger and vent rather than stew about it. I hold nothing in. If I do it makes me anxious. There was a time when I occasionally did frivolous shows, just to be funny: husband-and-wife competitions, battle of the sexes, what men think/what women think. But I stopped doing those kinds of shows because I don't have time to talk about stupid, silly things. Some of my producers tell me I've got to lighten up; I can't be too heavy every day. But most of the shows I do now are about major concerns. True crime. Death. Hate. I'll go home a wreck after talking to a little girl who had half her brain removed after being shot. But for most shows I try to leave how I feel at the office rather than bring that anxiety home.

There was one woman, however, a former supermodel named Karen Duffy, whose indomitable will against a truly despicable disease deeply affected me. She first came on my show on November 7, 2000, to talk about her book, *Model Patient: My Life As an Incurable Wise-Ass*. Karen had been one of *People* magazine's 50 Most Beautiful People in the World. She had been a veejay on MTV. And then she came down with sarcoidosis, a disease that's probably even tougher than MS. It started with a headache in the fall of 1995 and never subsided. It's like a tumor around the spinal cord. I saw a piece *Dateline* had done with her and I knew I had to talk to her, because I saw someone who was going through what I was—only the pain, fire and numbness I felt in my feet she felt all over her body. I can tell people that sometimes I feel as if I was standing naked and someone lit me on fire, but who can relate to that? Only someone else who actually knows what I'm describing. It's hard to imagine this beautiful young woman feels such fire and pain from head to toe. Her symptoms are similar to MS, but there is no remission, no relief.

Her neurologist told her she had a mostaccioli-sized lesion in her brain. It was like a penne noodle from her spinal column up into her medulla. She said when she heard this she was more ashamed than fearful. I understood completely—when I was first diagnosed, I, too, felt ashamed.

"It was growing," Karen told me. "It was damaging all the nerves that were talking to my body, so I lost feeling. It was just incredible pain. Imagine getting stung by a wasp, then by a jellyfish, then being set on fire—it's that sharp. And then it pulsates. I couldn't even wear clothes. I could not even move. I just laid in bed."

Karen spoke of the medicine she took to allow her to move and talk. It took her doctors eleven months before they figured out what she had was this rare disease of the central nervous system. It usually attacks lung tissue. In her case it attacked her brain and central nervous system. She was told to get her affairs in order. She received last rites. She underwent four and a half years of chemotherapy. And she survived to write her book and tell her story, even though she needs 200 milligrams of morphine just to put on a coat.

The thought of needing 200 milligrams of morphine just to make it through the day, every day, chilled me. It's shows like these that continue to put my life in perspective.

Those shows were all powerful examples of what television can do to educate and entertain. I've done shows about all the major news events of the past thirteen years. I didn't go to Oklahoma after the bombing of the Federal Building, but I had people from Oklahoma on the show. We had people on the show after the Columbine shootings; during the AIDS scare when a guy in upstate New York was going around trying to deliberately give people AIDS; the venereal disease outbreak in Mississippi. But they weren't the most powerful shows I've done. I'd have to say those that we did right after 9/11 were the ones I'll never forget.

I was doing a live satellite radio tour, where I speak to talk show hosts in different cities across the country every ten minutes for four hours promoting *The Montel Williams Show*. I was sitting in a small soundproof booth at CBS in New York talking to a DJ in Florida

about our eleventh season on the air when I glanced at a TV monitor
in the next room, where the technicians and some of my staff were.
That's when I saw the smoking hole where the first plane had entered
one of the World Trade Center buildings. I couldn't help letting out
an exclamation. The radio host in Florida was confused. "What?"

"Are you watching the news?" I said. "It looks like an airplane
just hit the World Trade Center." The disc jockey was speechless for
a second; then he said, "Montel, why don't you report it for us?" I
said, "I can't report it. I don't know anything. I'm sitting in a soundproof booth looking at a television screen."

The interview ended and it was time for my interview with a station in Ohio. The radio host said, "Montel, we heard what you just
said. We're changing the channels but there's nothing on the TV
here. What's going on?"

"It looks like a plane has just crashed into the World Trade Center," I said. "It's really strange though. I don't understand. . . ." And
then I let out the expletive "*Holy shit!*" As I watched, the second
plane had crashed into the other tower. "That was not a mistake!" I
yelled. "That plane deliberately flew into the building!"

The Ohio DJ saw what was happening on CNN and asked me to
do a blow-by-blow but I still couldn't hear the television. After a
minute I said to the DJ, "This is an inappropriate time for me to be
promoting *The Montel Williams Show*. We need to stop. I don't
know how many people have just lost their lives. . . ." We canceled
the rest of the radio promotions and watched in a daze as the smoke
poured out of the Twin Towers.

Out on the street, people were streaming out of buildings, not
sure where to go or how to get there, dialing useless cell phones over
and over, and looking south, always south, toward the burning towers at the foot of Manhattan. There was just this expression of dis-
belief on all the faces I saw. I considered trying to get out of the city
but decided that was not going to work because as I made my way
up to my office the city was becoming gridlocked.

After the second plane hit, I was not alone in thinking this had to
be a terrorist act; I wondered if we were under some sort of siege.
What would be the best course of action? Once I found out my chil-

dren were all safe, my thoughts focused on what I could do for the city. If I could get to my office I could start calling my producers to figure out what we were going to do. During that seemingly endless car ride my bodyguard Joe and I talked about how, when the World Trade Center had been attacked eight years earlier, I had mused that the best way to screw up America was to take those two buildings down. I figured you could shut down the economy immediately by dropping those buildings because you could kill 100,000 people at the same time and collapse the entire market—insurance companies and hospitals would go bankrupt. Was my nightmare scenario coming true?

In the time it took me to get back to the office through the choked streets, both towers had collapsed. I didn't envision those buildings imploding; I envisioned one of them falling into the other, which in turn would fall on top of others—that would have taken out seven blocks and an untold number of human lives. When they came down the way they did, with all the smoke and debris sucked in, I was horrified. How could people survive such a thing?

The city was understandably in chaos. All the bridges and tunnels were closed. The nation's airports were closed and all flights were canceled, so we certainly wouldn't be flying in any of our scheduled guests over the next few days. The regular show was clearly a lost cause. Since we tape ahead, we had two weeks' worth of shows ready to air, but our transmitter was located on top of the World Trade Center, so there wasn't going to be any *Montel Williams Show* in New York for a while. I wasn't really thinking about the show, anyway. Like any boss, I felt responsible for the people who worked for me, and I tried to be a calming presence. Then the Pentagon got hit—and I started to freak out. I had classmates down there! I immediately got on the phone and tried dialing everyone I knew, but all the phone lines were now shut down.

For two days you couldn't get clearance or permits to send a TV crew anywhere near Ground Zero. Emergency crews were reacting and responding. Rather than be like an ambulance chaser, I needed to give the city a chance to respond. I went back to my apartment, and from my window I could see a cloud coming up the Hudson River. It was a cloud of death permeating the city. The smell was worse than acrid animal flesh on the side of the road.

On Thursday I took a skeleton crew down to the site. We didn't know what kind of reception we would get from the firefighters and police and rescue workers—they had their hands more than full—but they were very helpful; they wanted the world to see what had happened. Anyone who was seeking access to the site had to go to a preauthorized location that the mayor and the police department set up to provide press credentials. That took two and a half hours. Once we got our credentials, we went to a media location that the police and fire departments had set up four or five blocks up the West Side Highway from where the World Trade Center had stood. From that spot they were taking groups of camera operators and reporters to within two blocks of the fallen towers. Truckloads of firefighters and rescue volunteers came in and out of that media location. I was able to interview on camera some of the people coming from Ground Zero. One of the emergency workers saw me and pinned an American flag on my back.

On Friday we found survivors who wanted to talk. I went to a hospital and spoke to a woman who had been an elevator operator in building two. She had been burned on her face and hands and was almost unrecognizable. Her husband was also an elevator operator and she thought he had died. She found out a few minutes before we showed up that her husband had survived and was at another hospital, but because of their injuries they couldn't get to each other. We orchestrated their reunion. It was phenomenal, and we later had them on our show to talk about their experiences. How many husband-and-wife teams were working that day in those buildings and survived? Here was one that did.

We edited the tapes we made and on Monday sent out the shows via satellite. They were heartfelt, powerful shows, but I wouldn't be surprised if no one saw them. Who was watching anything but the news for the next six months?

It was one thing for the nation to see that videotape of the planes crashing and the towers crumbling; it was another thing to be in lower Manhattan and see that pile of rubble and people screaming and crying and running everywhere trying to find survivors. It was an emotional cyclone and it sucked me right down. By Saturday morning I was in a bad way, shaking and shivering uncontrollably. It was hard to get up off the floor. I'm not sure if it was the chemicals that did it or the emotion, but 9/11 set off a flare-up, no question. The pain was incredible. The ground poured forth such a savage dust from the disintegrated dead flesh and compressed debris that were once those twin towers that it affected me for weeks afterward. But what was going on with me seemed so insignificant compared to what other people had been through. Joe had seen me coughing and struggling to breathe when we were down there doing our interviews and he asked how I was doing. I said I was okay but I was lying. I knew it truly did mess with me but I was praying it was something that wasn't going to last.

Maybe it wasn't smart of me to go down there, but what else could I do? I wasn't thinking about the smells or what breathing that polluted air might do to exacerbate my MS. All I knew was that I had to get these stories out. I don't know if that was smart but it was the only honest reaction I could have had.

9

I'm a Sexual Being

I have this habit, whenever I can't sleep, of getting into my Prowler and cruising around the city. I remember this one beautiful night the week before 9/11, around one or two in the morning, I had the top down and was doing my usual loop. I drove down to Battery Park, cut in front of the World Trade Center to look up at those giant skyscrapers touching the moon, then screamed back up the West Side Highway to Thirty-fourth Street, then up Eighth Avenue to Lincoln Center before making a left on Sixty-sixth Street and returning home. Whenever I stopped at a light, people who were still hanging at that hour of the morning would flick me a grin and say, "What's up, dog? How you doin', man?"

A few days after 9/11 I wasn't feeling well and probably like the rest of the city I couldn't sleep, so I got into the Prowler to do my loop and take my mind off things. But this time I couldn't cut in front of those twin towers, couldn't get anywhere near where they once stood. I could only smell the foul air and think of all the people who lost their lives and how fragile we are—and not just those of us who lived in Manhattan, but all of us. I thought about my staff and the people they were mourning; about the show and the pressure we would be under to come up with a meaningful response.

Just two weeks earlier I had been snowboarding in Chile. I don't quite understand why being on a snowboard brings my pain down from a nine to a two, but it does. Somehow the way my brain is wired, when I get on that board my feet are sending SOS signals up through my scarred nerves that actually get through. So when I returned, right before those two planes changed our world, I was feeling pretty good.

When the tragedy hit I heard from Grace. We didn't get along and rarely spoke, other than coordinating seeing the children and such. Now she had a new boyfriend and his mother was staying in a hotel down near Ground Zero. She wanted to know if I would help this woman get out of town. So I sent a car for her and got the lady out of the city. September 11 helped Grace and me put aside some of the pettiness we had come to think of as the norm.

It wasn't just our relationship; the magnitude of the tragedy put *everything* into a different perspective. And when I reevaluated my life, the one thing I kept coming back to was love. Women have always been important to me, and when you get a vision of war and the devastation of a city—which is what happened to those of us who lived in New York—you begin to think about the important things in life. And I don't care who you are, when it comes to thinking like this what you think about is love.

If love is lacking in your life, as it was for me, then you might also think about sex.

Human beings are sexual beings. But for me, it's always been more. Sex has been my gauge, my proof that I'm okay, that I'm worthy. My first sexual experience was when I was twelve. The girl was fourteen. We were at her house. We kissed. I was playing with her. She was playing with me. Did I have any knowledge of what I was doing? Hell, no. Did I think what I was doing was sex? No, it was just something that felt good. That's what started me off because I was the only kid in my neighborhood who got a little experience. From that point on I attempted to do it with every girl I knew. When I was around fourteen, the heavy petting started, but my first experience with sexual intercourse was when I was fifteen . . . and the girl got pregnant. I went with her to a clinic and she had an abortion. It cost three hundred dollars and was a traumatic and emotional experience for both of us. We attempted to handle it matter-of-factly, but two weeks later we sat down and cried about it. It hit us both that we were going to have a child and we just killed that child. No one ever knew.

Soon after I went to Denmark on an exchange program called People-to-People. An eighteen-year-old Danish girl tried her best to instruct me in every facet of sexuality. I was in seventh heaven. I came back from Denmark a changed man! I'd decided I would only go out with older girls. I was like the stud of studs. In my senior year a teacher's aide, who had already been under investigation for sleeping with a student, took me home and we had a hot affair for four weeks, until we got caught and she got fired. She was twenty-six. They called my mother about it but otherwise hushed it up. I was a black kid being bussed to a school for integration; she was a white teacher's aide and no one wanted this out.

The next couple of years, in the early seventies, I was running around with girls everywhere. I ended up having to deal with three more abortions. I have no idea why I was not more careful—I was as stupid as stupid could be. I was seventeen the second time; the third time we were both in the marines; the fourth I was at the Naval Academy. That last one, she didn't want the abortion, but I talked her into it. That was the one that sent me over the edge. From that point on I stopped running around and started going with one person at a time, making sure we always used birth control.

While stationed in Guam I met the woman who would become my first wife. I asked her to marry me a month and a half after we met because I was having paternal feelings and I did not want to go through any more abortions. I wanted to be a father because I felt like I'd destroyed so many previous opportunities. We were married for eight years, and suffice it to say we were on opposite ends of the sexual spectrum. She was dealing with some issues from her childhood that prohibited her from having an open sex life and I was coming from having an abundant sex life. So we clashed.

I didn't become aware of my sexual anomalies until I was in my mid-thirties and a talk show host. That's when things started getting strange. I might have sex five days in a row and the next day not be able to ejaculate at all. I thought it was a psychological issue. I went to a therapist about it and was told I was just getting older, but I didn't buy that. I thought it was either the anxiety of entering into a new relationship or the fear of having a child that was stopping me from ejaculating. The truth is I should have been checked for MS.

Then I married Grace. We produced two wonderful children and I think she would agree that we had a good sex life, but at the same time we had multiple occasions to talk about my sexual anomalies. We might be getting ready to be intimate and I'm not there. Five minutes after we stop I'm there for the next forty-five minutes. Hello?

* * *

That's the way it's been. It's not an ego thing; it's just that in my low of lows it can make me feel whole to have someone hold me, someone who has obviously enjoyed me. It was always this way, but especially since my diagnosis. In some way I think I felt that I had to overcompensate. But I also know it's part of who I am to seek affirmation in sex.

And as the saying goes, seek and ye shall find.

Dr. Counter had once teased me about finding a nice Swedish woman; little did I know that I would! On the night before I left Sweden in December 1998, I met a wonderful woman named Mia.* She reminded me of Ingrid Bergman in every way: in person, in beauty, in grace, in style. We talked, and kissed, and I told her that I was in the process of getting divorced but that when I was legally separated I'd be fair game.

I called her many times after my return to New York. We'd talk for hours and I was amazed at how freely we could share everything. I told her about my illness and my suicide attempts, and she shared painful things about her own life. I went back to see her in February and we took a romantic trip to Paris and Amsterdam. We walked along the Champs-Élysées; we ate in four-star restaurants; we took boat rides along the canals in Amsterdam, and visited the van Gogh Museum. We were spending our nights together but not attempting to be intimate with each other. We were getting to know each other and taking it slow. One of the things I remember thinking was that she was someone who would feel more bound to respect the bonds of marriage in sickness and in health. That was a big thing for me as I started to get to know her. But while I was surprisingly honest with her about what I was going through, I was still internalizing a good deal. I was afraid to confess my fears or to complain about my pain.

That's just how it had been with Grace. We who suffer from MS often don't treat our spouses or loved ones correctly. We don't want to become a burden, so we don't share our powerful, sometimes

*Names have been changed for privacy considerations.

scary feelings. If you don't have a really solid relationship then you're definitely not going to share things, but unfortunately if you're not sharing it's going to make your relationship worse. That's what happened with Grace and me. We weren't on solid footing to begin with, and my fear of opening up to someone who I didn't trust would be there for me really undermined my ability to communicate, which caused even more problems.

Perhaps that's why I felt that Mia could not have come into my life at a more perfect time or been a more perfect respite for me.

I didn't realize it at the time, but ever since my diagnosis a year earlier I had been out to prove that I was okay sexually. To me it was simply a benchmark, if not of health, then of normalcy. So once we got past the getting-to-know-you stage, sex became a large part of our relationship. Mia was fifteen years younger than I, and Northern European to boot. European women have a more open attitude toward sex. For them it's about taking time and making love, as compared to many American women who just want to do it and get on with other things. I had a wonderful sexual relationship with Mia because she enjoyed it as much as I did. It seemed that everywhere we went we were having sex. Outside, inside, on airplanes, wherever.

She flew to New York in April, stayed a while, went back, and then returned and stayed for three months. And boy, when she moved in, she moved in! The girl was repainting my apartment, redecorating, pulling stuff down. I'd go to work and come home and everything was changed. I told her to have fun during the day and she did!

Mia was up for anything and everything. We had a great relationship, going places and doing things. We went snowboarding in Canada, to the beach in Florida, hung out in L.A. She accompanied me to the Carousel Ball in Los Angeles and the Angel Ball in New York. We were almost inseparable. The kids got along with her wonderfully; it was incredible to see Wyntergrace and Gooch hugging her and laughing with her.

It was all fantastic. Mia was ready to get married and have babies. I thought, great, for that she would love and take care of me. I was running right down the aisle to get married when I realized, hold on,

I just got divorced! I'm not really ready to get married again! And I wasn't sure about having babies. Because of the drugs I was taking, I went to a fertility doctor to see if I would be capable of having more children. The answer was basically "Hell, no." The chances are just too great that any child conceived with me would have some birth defect. So I can't have any more kids. The harsh reality of all those drugs in my system and my age truly set in. I was not going to be Richard Gere, at the age of fifty with a one-year-old.

It came to a head in December 1999 when for visa reasons she had to go back to Sweden for at least a month. I could have married her, or I could have bought some time by bringing her back as a nanny for eighteen months, but I said no, it was time to end it. Would she not have been the perfect mate? Probably. At least she was the type of person who'd have stuck with me through thick and thin. But I wasn't ready to commit for a lifetime. And there was that issue of kids.

My assistant packed up all evidence of her existence in my apartment, five boxes' worth, and sent them to her via FedEx. We didn't speak for two months, and when we finally did it didn't go well.

In the year after that I went out with several women, and with each one it was different. But all of it was stressful, because when you're intimate with someone, she naturally wants to know more about you, and there's something about this disease that makes you not want to open up. I had no choice, sometimes. If my body wasn't functioning normally, I had to say something. How would you like to be a guy saying, "I'll make love to you but unfortunately I can't come," or "You know, funny thing: sometimes I require a lot of foreplay to get an erection, and other times it's normal"?

Believe me, I'd rather not have to go into why my body acts the way it does—it just brings me down. And it's not just in the bedroom. I might go to a movie and have to excuse myself to go to the bathroom the second the movie starts. Same thing at a restaurant. Obviously the lady is going to be wondering, waiting for an explanation, when I really don't feel like talking about it! But sex is the worst. I don't want to feel embarrassed, but society has made me embarrassed; we're taught to believe that if we don't act like the 1 percent of the population that has the perfect orgasm then obviously we're screwed up. It's estimated that 60 percent of all men over the age of twenty-five have experienced some sort of erectile dysfunction. And yet each of us feels inadequate!

The truth is what we eat, how we exercise, what we weigh, how we worry, how many times we masturbate—all these things affect us as we get older. And MS affects the nerves in my body—sometimes I feel pain, sometimes I feel nothing. I could make love for a long time without feeling anything. And there is nothing anyone can do.

Before I was diagnosed these same things happened but I had no explanation for them. I just thought they were psychological. After my diagnosis I started reading about the ways MS affects men sexually.

But the truth is, sexual anomalies don't occur only with those of us who have MS. The drugs people take for high blood pressure, diabetes, Parkinson's, or extreme sinus issues can cause the same problems. There are something like 30 million prescriptions a year being written for Viagra. That's a whole lot of guys having some problems that aren't being discussed.

In America sexuality seems to be divided into foreplay, intercourse, orgasm. When you start interacting with other cultures you realize it's way broader than that. Intimacy is much broader. It's not just foreplay—it's conversation, and holding.

I am a sexual being even with the issues I have. It may not be perfect all the time, but it's always an incredible experience in spite of any annoying anomalies.

In January 2000 I saw a striking dark-haired woman in my audience and wound up dating her for two months. Her name was Cathy and she was a terrific lady, but I knew it wasn't going to work in the long run because I wasn't willing to commit to someone with children. In my mind I felt that I had become a burden to my own children, and I didn't want to extend that to someone else's.

It was around this time I started having tremendous problems with my skin. Certain parts of my body became unbearably sensitive; if I was touched in those places it could make me jump across the room. One is a circular patch four inches from my belly button. If someone touches me there it sends a pain right through my stomach to my spine. It can be as light as a breeze, as light as a dust particle falling from the ceiling over my bed and landing on my naked belly. It's not that extreme all the time but it's there every second of the day.

This symptom has been unbelievably depressing. You don't realize how often people touch you. Especially as a celebrity—guys who greet you don't just say, "Hey, how ya doin'?" They've got to add a *smack!* They have to hit you on the back or the shoulder. I don't know why—it's something in a man's nature. There are days when I can take that but there are days when I feel like knocking somebody down. Not long ago I got into a packed elevator, and a woman had a purse that was pressing up against my back. That did it for me and elevators. I can't get in a crowded elevator now because I'm afraid someone will accidentally brush against me and make me jump or flinch.

So imagine how it is with a person I care about. I really have to try my best to suppress jumping away because I know that would be insulting! I don't want to turn someone off by making her feel bad. So I try my best to fight the urge to recoil. And yet we all require touch. Look at what happens to babies raised in orphanages who are put in cribs and never touched—they wind up having all kinds of developmental issues. I need closeness and intimacy as much as anyone else. I want to be touched! But there are times when I just can't be, and that drives me crazy.

The next woman I went out with after Cathy was a professional masseuse. How's that for irony? I met her while on a snowboarding vacation in Utah, and as long as she avoided my numb spots, her vigorous touch was soothing.

Then I met Sarah, also in Utah. She looked like a pinup model and she had a G-string tattoo on her body. I like girls with ink! We had a lot of fun, but another disturbing symptom arose.

One night right in the midst of making love, I had this big flash of pain that felt like it was shooting right out of the head of my penis. The pain ran up my leg through my testicles and out my penis.

"Hold on a second," I said through clenched teeth. "We gotta stop."

"Why?" she asked.

All I could say was "Please." And I rolled over and eased her off of me.

She could see from my face that something was very wrong. There was no dodging this one. I told her what had happened, and she was as loving and nice and sweet as she could be. It was one of the more intimate moments of my adult life, because she was not just trying to be understanding—she was trying to understand. I had to get up and go into the bathroom for a minute and cry. I was crying because of the pain and the disappointment. First, I hurt and I had to stop because the more I attempted to have sex the more I hurt. That triggered the emotional outburst. What was a wonderful moment had turned into one where I couldn't be touched. I felt I'd let her down. And then I felt, why can't this stop? I tried to use my visualization technique to put my pain in the box, but on this night it wouldn't go. All I could do was lie with my arm around her until the morning, which drove me crazy.

I felt like I had failed. It wasn't so much the sex as it was the amplification that I'm ill and there is something wrong. I talked to one urologist about it and he said, "Man, you're forty-five years old. What are you complaining about? A lot of guys can't even have sex." Okay, great; thanks—not exactly the answer I was looking for!

My next serious relationship lasted two years, until the spring of 2003. Tina was a model from Winnipeg, Canada, and an extraordinary spirit. I fell completely in love with her and will probably love her until the day I die.

Winnipeg has a large cluster of people with MS, so she was aware of the disease, and when we started seeing each other she got in touch with her aunt, who was a nurse, and learned how to give me my shots. She studied and read everything she could about MS. I felt that she had made a conscious decision to be with me, and that no matter what happened she would be there.

We exchanged every vow of love we could. I went out and bought her an engagement ring. And in the end, she broke up with me and I still haven't gotten over it. I am still trying to figure it out.

There were a lot of mitigating circumstances. In our two-year relationship I had violated a trust one time, and though it wasn't what I considered the most egregious offense, it was something she could never forgive me for; and for that I shall forever pay the price of losing one of the true treasures of my life. Along with this she had been in the midst of a never-ending divorce and I was probably the perfect transitional relationship for her. In the end we broke up, I believe, for as many reasons as there were no reasons at all.

But one thing has haunted me, one thing that in hindsight seems like the crux of the problem. We took a trip to Europe for my birthday, which was great fun until we boarded a plane from Amsterdam to New York, with a stopover in Paris. Fifteen minutes into the flight I started to shake. My temperature rose to 102. By the time we reached Charles de Gaulle Airport I could barely walk.

We immediately got the Concorde back to New York because there was no way I wanted to deal with my medical problems in an unfamiliar place. I was sweating and shivering all the way back. The next day I went to see my doctor. He confirmed that I had the flu and that my fever had brought out my symptoms. I was dehydrated and he gave me two bags of IV fluids. I felt really sick, coughing and sneezing, sensitive to touch, my feet on fire. For two miserable days I thought I was done; some doctors think that during a fever we develop new lesions.

Instead of being supportive, Tina surprised me by being angry. "You don't even take the time to take care of your MS!" she said. In her eyes I had been neglecting myself because I hadn't gone to Sweden to see Dr. Olsson or to Harvard for a checkup. But here's the thing: that didn't mean I wasn't taking care of myself. In fact, that was exactly what I was doing: taking care of myself, by myself. I was following my medication and exercise regimen completely, trying my best to lessen my stress. She was worried for me, because I hadn't been completely open about all the aspects of my disease. I hadn't let her completely in.

I despise feeling vulnerable. I disdain it. I hate it.

I hate it when a woman runs her knee down my calf and I shoot off of the bed because it feels so bad when, before this disease, it used to feel so good.

I hate having to worry before making love to a woman whether the pain will set in, or my penis will change its mind. I hate it when I cannot beat the pain. When I can't function. When I don't want to talk about it. When everything is so messed up that I sometimes become nasty. When I can't take a shower because the water hurts my skin. When the breeze from an air purifier makes me anxious. I hate it when by the end of the day I have more cramps than when the day began.

And I hate it when I wake up in the morning and lie to myself about the day before because I know I'm going to try to hide any residual pain left over.

What I have been hiding because of this illness has been the lowest self-esteem I've ever felt in my life. I'm at the bottom of the barrel. I've been there and I'm still here. Because I feel like I can't do what I used to be able to do—from untroubled sex to walking to running. I'm working very hard at lifting myself out of that hole, even though I sometimes feel like I don't deserve to get out. But it's this internal battle that helps to motivate me because I refuse to allow myself to stay at the bottom of the well; it's part of the essence of who I am and why I continue to try my best and why I'm not going to let this disease get the best of me.

I'd like to think that MS had nothing to do with the breakup of my last relationship, but it did. MS has been a barrier in *every* relationship I've had.

People with MS need to make a huge effort to bring people into our world. We tell people what's wrong only when we feel like telling them, and then we stop. It becomes this dance of double-talk rather than just trying to tell the truth. I think more marriages would be preserved if people were 100 percent open about the disease from the beginning, rather than taking months to get to the same point, after the damage has already been done. Otherwise, the spouse feels left out, like you're closing up and you're pushing them away. It's part of the reason a lot of people with MS end up divorced. If you are in a relationship where you are used to sharing your emotions and all of a sudden you get this disease and you shut down, you are taking something away from your spouse. And your spouse is going to notice, and naturally feel rejected.

I did this with Grace. I've done something of the same thing with other women, sharing just so much and no more. I've told them I have MS and what it is, but that doesn't truly explain it. How can you tell someone you're just getting to know that she may one day find you jumping away from her when the pain comes on? You can't. So you stay quiet, hoping it won't happen. And when it does, it scares them. That's why so many people who have MS end up alone. We are so afraid to tell the truth to those people around us because of the fear of rejection. All you need is one person to reject you and that can set the course for the rest of your life.

There's a line in a song by 50 Cent: "It's easy to love me now, would you love me if I was down and out?" It's a lot easier to love me while I look good, but what about when I start getting sicker? The question has to be asked while I'm still in relatively good shape. That's one of the insidious things about this disease. You can look good but not feel well.

Ever since I became a celebrity I've had to wonder if someone likes me for me or because I'm well known; when she got to know the real me, not the TV personality, would she still like me? Now the real me is sick, vulnerable; who could possibly love that person?

I'm feeling extremely jaded about relationships, extremely wary. I'm almost afraid to walk down that path right now because I'm a little distrusting. I find it very hard to accept a compliment. I see what's wrong rather than what's right in me. And what's wrong is that I have multiple sclerosis.

I might find someone who will stick with me for a long period of time, I might even find someone to marry, but I can no longer look at life and think about a lifelong relationship. I wish I could, but I just don't believe it can happen to me anymore.

10

Screaming with Joy at the Top of My Lungs

If there's been any consistency in my life over the last twenty-five years it's been in the attention I've paid to keeping my body fit. I've been active in sports from the time I was a child. I was a three-letter athlete in high school; I played JV basketball, football and track. I studied martial arts under three different instructors, and earned green belts and brown belts. I also sang in a band and dressed like Jimi Hendrix—open vests with midriff shirts—and to pull that off, I needed six-pack abs. So I was always exercising, hitting a speed bag, doing calisthenics and push-ups. When I was younger I had a hard time putting on weight; I was one of them skinny-as-a-rail kids. I admired people who went to the gym and pumped. I went and pumped and nothing happened. But I kept doing it because it was about the building. Then in the marine corps and at the Naval Academy I continued to work on my body. It became an integral part of my life. I went from entering the service at 145 pounds, boxing as a welterweight, to 180 pounds of solid muscle. I maintained a perfect rating on the PFT (physical fitness test) throughout my years in the service. When I went to Guam, I took third place in the Mr. Guam bodybuilder competition and won Best Poser. That's the shape I've attempted to keep myself in, a competitive athletic level. Being physically fit makes a difference in the way people react to you. If you walk into a room full of naval officers and you are in the best shape, it gives you a psychological edge over your peers. Did I use that to my advantage in situations where race could be an issue? Absolutely. Very seldom does a redneck jump up in the face of somebody who could beat him down. It's just that simple. The muscles I have now at my age are the residual effect of all the hard work I've put in over the years. That attention broke down for eight months after my diagnosis, but I know that the one thing that has kept me physically doing all the things I do is my workout regimen. I'm in the gym by seven every morning doing resistance training and aerobics.

Before my diagnosis I worked out more for solid bulk strength, pushing as much weight as I could. I used to deadlift 585 pounds.

I first began looking for a trainer to work out with while I was doing the dramatic series *Matt Waters* in December 1994. In one of the episodes the first scene called for me to jump into a pool in a bathing suit. I had two weeks to get myself ready to take my clothes off. I saw Wini Linguvic, a highly sought-out personal trainer, working with people in the World Gym at Sixty-fourth and Broadway. I was in strength and bulk mode and had not concentrated at all on physique for a long time. I asked Wini to help me out. For the next two weeks she pounded me. I really liked the way she trained—she showed me that I could get into camera-ready shape in that short time—and wanted to continue working with her. But she had too many clients at the time and pointed me toward Ritchie, a friend of hers. I wanted to go back to strength training and Ritchie was a good strength trainer who had worked with one of the U.S. Olympic team trainers. So I worked out with Ritchie from 1995 until a week before my diagnosis in 1998. At that time I was deadlifting 425 pounds off the rack. I was squatting 350 pounds. Bench-pressing 300.

As soon as I got diagnosed I called Ritchie and said, "I was wondering if I could hire you away from your entire training practice?" I offered to pay him full salary just to manage my physical fitness health care. But he wanted to get out of personal training, so he suggested that I ask Wini. She had way too many clients for me to ask her to give them up, so I asked instead if she would make me a priority and train me every day.

We started training and Wini and I just clicked. Not only is she in ridiculously good shape, but I love that she's a pragmatic, no-nonsense trainer. She's also a physical therapist who was able to understand MS and design a workout specifically for my symptoms—for example, changing around exercises to work on my balance. We evolved the idea of getting fit for life rather than just fit for a limited objective, such as when I was working out to look good in photos or to increase the amount of weight I could lift. Fitness for life is about achieving a level of physical fitness that allows you to meet any life challenge head-on. And for me that means to face the challenge of my MS.

I can go into that gym feeling awful, walking badly, having difficulty making it up that flight of stairs, and after our workout I will bounce out with a smile on my face. Then there have been days I've been hurting and I've gone to the gym and hid in a corner, just hugging Wini, because I feel so bad. She helps me get through it. I've cried with her more than once. Wini has been one of those voices that remind me that I need to stay on track.

Although looking good wasn't the point of the program we developed, it had the side benefit of giving me a better physique. People in the gym were constantly coming up and asking us questions about what we were doing. For three weeks I would do regular sets; for the next three weeks I would do supersets (two exercises back-to-back with no break). Then the next three weeks I would do giant sets (three exercises back-to-back). People who watched me thought I looked like the Tasmanian devil. I'd be smokin', doing one hundred sets an hour, more than one set per minute. Once in that groove I'd be dripping sweat and pounding. And the results were obvious.

So we decided to coauthor a book called *BodyChange: The 21-Day Fitness Program for Changing Your Body . . . and Your Life!* We thought it would help people understand that no matter what shape you are in, even if you have a chronic illness, you can still work out. Eventually I'd like to be able to design an entire course of rehabilitative exercise with equipment that will fine-tune the way people who are differently abled train and stay in shape.

As heartened as I am that I can still lift weights and that people compliment me on my physique and strength, the truth is I've gotten weaker in the last five years. I haven't attempted to deadlift over 300 pounds since I've been ill and don't know if I could now. That's almost half of what I could do when I was forty-two. For me that's devastating. My age has nothing to do with it. Men can maintain their strength until they are in their mid-sixties. There are sixty-year-old guys in my gym who can bench-press 400 pounds. But you know, I'm also reminded every day that I am still blessed with the ability to walk into that gym, so I'll get used to leaving my ego at the door and be proud of the fact that I can still lift something.

Remember the story of Samson and Delilah? When Delilah cut

Samson's hair, he lost his strength; he wasn't Samson anymore. That's how I sometimes feel. I'm not Samson anymore; it's gone. I cannot get on the treadmill and run for six miles in the morning like I used to. Not only that, but going on the treadmill has become painfully embarrassing because of the awkward way I walk. But Wini has convinced me I have to do it anyway. So I get on the treadmill and wonder if people in that gym are watching me walk the way I do.

If people are going to watch me do something, I'd prefer it be how I snowboard.

It was Guy Rocourt who got me into snowboarding. Guy was the first assistant director on *Little Pieces* and we spent hours and hours working on the movie together. Sometimes Gooch would come and play video games on the set. His favorite was one about snowboarding and he was always saying, "Daddy, I want to go snowboarding." Because of my illness I didn't think I could do it. Guy had been snowboarding for five years so we talked about it. I told him about the pain and numbness in my ankles and feet; how I'd trip going up the stairs because I couldn't tell how high to lift my feet; how I at times stumble just getting up from my desk because my feet don't feel the floor.

"Snowboarding might help," Guy said. "You'll never know if you don't try."

What did I have to lose? Gooch wanted to learn, Guy was experienced; if I couldn't do it, I'd hang around and look at the women. So after I returned from my first trip to Sweden we went to Park City, Utah, and I learned to snowboard.

It wasn't easy. At first, I got trashed. It hurt. Gooch took some lessons, but I figured Guy could guide me, so I just went out with him. I got on that board and I slapped my ass to the ground about sixty times before getting to the first chairlift. Getting on the chairlift wasn't difficult, but getting off was; I was thrown right to the ground and smashed my face. Then I must have fallen thirty times on my way down to the bottom of the first hill. I was a buffoon. But I was determined to learn how to snowboard—after all, I had already invested $500 in boots and jackets and another $400 for the board!

Guy did his best to help me find my footing—literally. "You're attempting to force the board to do what it can't do; you need to try to ride on one edge or the other."

On the plus side, snowboarding was different from skiing. In skiing your legs are independent, and because my left leg is slightly weaker than my right, I'm afraid of breaking my weaker leg. But in snowboarding your feet are locked together and together they move one object. My right leg could therefore compensate for my weaker left leg.

There are times when I am looking straight ahead and I don't know where the floor is; or I'm climbing stairs and I can't tell where the next step is. I literally don't know where my feet are. At times I feel like I am walking on my ankles, like there is nothing underneath them. It's one of my great frustrations, and yet, after snowboarding awhile, I was able to feel where my feet were. Maybe it had to do with the tight boots, which helped make me aware of my feet, or the fact that the boots were locked into a set of bindings, which means my feet were always in the same place, where my brain would recognize them. Even if I fell, my feet were still in the bindings. I knew where they were! If my brain sent a signal to curl my toes, it actually happened. For someone who often doesn't know where his feet are, this is reason enough to keep snowboarding. If I fall it's not because of MS, it's because I made a mistake, just like anyone else. I'm functioning normally.

To say I was accosted by the snow that first day is an understatement. On the second day I was brutally mugged. It took me two hours to do one run that would now take me five minutes. By the third day, I'd taken some bad falls, including colliding with a skier who was coming down a nonmarked trail and didn't give me the right-of-way. My knees and shoulder were swollen. My feet were burning from being locked into the boots for four hours. I was wiped out. Gooch, on the other hand, at all of five years old, was sticking to the board and going down the hill like a rocket. By the end of the weekend he was able to come to a perfect stop on one edge.

I figured as long as I didn't break anything the knocks were well worth what I was getting out of it, because by the end of the weekend the fire in my feet was starting to subside, and I could also do something in spite of my MS.

When I told Dr. Olek about snowboarding, he was surprised. He said sports like that could be dangerous because a lot of people with MS have poor coordination and unpredictable spasms. If you had a spasm while snowboarding, you might seriously hurt yourself.

I understood his concern, but I also knew that my brain was working differently when I snowboarded, and that my feet were responding in ways they hadn't since being diagnosed. That's what drove me to go again two weekends later, and from that point forward I went every single weekend until the end of the ski season. I had been snowboarding for thirty-seven days. Unfortunately, I didn't take a lesson until about the twentieth day.

What a mistake! I don't care what kind of ego you have or what you've done before; *you need to take a lesson* from somebody who understands the principles of falling down a mountain on a piece of wood or plastic. If I had known what this sport was all about I would have first used a balance board, which was developed to help skateboarders train, or at least had someone show me the proper stance and go over some basic technique. If I had left my ego at the door, I sure would have saved myself a mess of bruises.

I kept going back to Park City once a month and eventually rented a house in Utah. There are eleven mountains within easy distance of Salt Lake City where you can snowboard. Different resorts, different terrain, different areas of the state. Utah, however, is not a very popular place with brothers. There are certain places in this country where people of color are routinely not seen and therefore we are ignored. And there are other places, like certain resorts, where it feels like an alarm goes off when a black person drives up. Everybody stares. They want you to feel uncomfortable. They're not used to seeing people of color on mountains and they make sure you know that. There are several places around America like that, where racist people go on their vacations to get away from people of color. They'll walk by your table and look you up and down like, what are *you* doing here? I run into people in lift lines who huff and puff and make comments about black people being there.

When we first went to Park City, Guy and I were the only two black people on that entire mountain. I almost had to deck a guy behind us who felt he needed to use the N word to let us know he knew we were there: "I've been on this mountain for five years. I ain't never seen niggers out here and all of a sudden they're here all the time." You even get it from a few employees out there. The ski industry has a long way to go to attract minorities!

Most of the people I get looks from are my age or older; thankfully it's almost the opposite with the youth of America. Kids come up to me all the time who clearly don't know who I am; they're just psyched to see a black guy snowboarding. "Yo, what's up, dude? Great board, man. Where you from? That's so cool, man. We don't see a lot of brothers up here. . . ." White kids actually say things like that. Hip-hop has become pop culture and that transcends race and economics.

By my second year with the sport Guy and I had snowboarded in Mammoth, in Squaw Valley, in Whistler, Lake Louise and Mount Tremblant up in Canada; we'd traveled to the Italian Alps and Chile. We were always in search of fresh snow. If I was only snowboarding twelve or twenty days a year then one resort would be fine, but I do four or five times that. And wherever I go, I'll do fifteen to twenty runs in a day. If I just stayed in Utah, it wouldn't be as challenging. What makes you good is being able to do it anywhere, in any kind of conditions. I want to be able to be dropped off by helicopter in Alaska and take a seventeen-mile ride.

To be able to ride a snowboard in powder takes some skill. When you find a patch of powder that you can sink into and ride, it's like being on a magic carpet. It's like what you see in a cartoon: Aladdin on the carpet floating in the air; his body is still but that carpet is just rippling below. Riding fresh soft snow you can feel your snowboard rippling beneath you or else it's like smoothly cutting through butter. Your upper body is still and it feels like there is nothing below you, like you're riding on air. The sensation of the ride clearly registers in my head. As I sail down that mountain, all doubts go away and I feel like I can do just about anything.

And I do it with friends who are some of the craziest people I know, friends who do risky, dumb jumps and turns, and I'll go right along with them. We'll go up and down on the lift until we've worn out the snow; then we'll go jumping off the trail and board clear around to the other side of the mountain. At the Canyon Resort in

Park City I've ridden eleven chairlifts in three hours. With snow-boarding, it's all about testosterone: we're all busting each other about who can do something better. It's hysterical. I'm forty-seven years old and I can put my daughter's friends off the mountain. By three p.m. they're ready to quit but they don't because the old man is still raring to go. That charges me up!

I also snowboard with my friend Jama Anderson, a certified instructor who keeps me out of trouble. With her it's not about ego or trying to beat each other, like with some of the guys; it's just about riding and having fun. She's very talented, so most of the time we let Jama pick the line and just follow her. There was one jump we wanted to do in Chile but it looked too dangerous; none of the guys wanted to test it first, so we called Jama and she did it. To call Jama extreme is an understatement.

Women are just great snowboarders. They move their hips and ankles in a way most guys don't. Men should really watch and try to mimic the motion. That rhythm is what you need to ride a snowboard.

I've enjoyed skydiving out of airplanes, in-line skating, surfing . . . but I feel most alive when I'm snowboarding, when I'm on the top of a mountain. On that board I'm charged. I don't care if people look at me as I go down a mountain—with all my gear on they don't even know it's me most of the time. I can scream with joy at the top of my lungs from riding through a patch of powder that is four inches deep.

I am in the best mood when I wake up at the crack of dawn, look out the back window of my house in Utah and see new snow on the mountain, knowing that I will be riding down it after breakfast.

Before I started snowboarding the feeling that my feet had disap-peared was happening every day. Two days of snowboarding gives me five days of feet. Five days of snowboarding gives me fifteen days of feet. If I'm on my board for three or four days at a time I can reduce my pain from a nine to a two. I walk better, I climb stairs bet-ter, and I feel almost normal. I'll go to the ends of the earth with my snowboard to feel that way. Even if it's only temporary.

I hope that one day it's no longer temporary. When I retire I will chase snow around this planet all year round and I'll feel good. Period.

11

In the First Grade, Anticipating Graduation!

The more I think about multiple sclerosis, the more I realize what a strange disease it is. In 1986 we didn't know any more about it than we did in 1836. That's because doctors could never come to definite conclusions about it. They didn't know what caused it. They didn't know how to treat it. They didn't realize that if you lost your vision or had pain in your feet or numbness in your arms or felt run-down to the point of being bedridden for days it was because your immune system was wreaking havoc on your nervous system.

Now we know that MS causes some form of signal degradation between the brain and various parts and organs in the body. We know that as the disease progresses, each time you go into an episode or a bout you will likely come out with some new scarring or degradation. Sometimes that scarring takes place in an area of the brain that has a very palpable effect on the body and sometimes it causes no symptoms. Even more oddly, the same place I have a scar may manifest symptoms differently in someone else than it does in me. That's just the nature of MS.

There are core symptoms that maybe 60 percent of MS patients have. The rest of us may have symptoms that no one else we know has. That's what's so tough about the disease and why it's so hard for doctors to home in on a cure. I have twenty-seven scars on my brain and spinal cord; another person with that many may not be able to walk.

What is it that we really know about MS today? If you polled ten of America's top scientists who are respected throughout the world for their acumen as neurologists and as MS specialists, you'd probably come away with six different answers to that question. (Some doctors do agree!) This is what makes it so incredibly hard on all of us who suffer. We don't know what to read or what to believe. If the doctors who have been studying this disease can't agree, then what am I supposed to think?

I wanted to be able to present the most up-to-the-minute information available, so as an appendix I've asked seven of the leading doctors in the field to answer questions that have been touched upon throughout this book, and some that haven't but should be answered. I don't agree with some of their responses, but that's okay. I've never agreed with all the things doctors have told me.

That's why I believe it's important for all of us to be our own detectives, investigators and researchers. We have to individually experiment, take a look to see what we are allergic to; see what exacerbates our disease or any one of our symptoms and work to alleviate that.

In the last twenty years we have bridged a gap that for more than one hundred fifty years we couldn't come anywhere near closing. And in the last five years we have really started to break this disease apart. Hopefully in the next two years we are going to identify what MS truly is.

What I think we know so far about MS is that the disease appears to be one of the autoimmune system. For some reason the immune system is treating the T3/T4 protein as a foreign body and attacking it in our myelin. That's the theory behind the MS drug Copaxone: to trick the immune system into thinking the drug is the foreign agent it should be attacking instead. In contrast, the theory behind Avonex and Betaseron is to try to modify the immune system.

I'm taking MS drug therapy on faith that it is actually slowing down my disease and reducing the number of bouts, but frankly there is no proof. There is not enough data on any of the current drugs because the disease goes in cycles. The drugs have been in use about ten years, and we really won't know if they work until they've been in use at least twenty. I just hope three years from now somebody doesn't come along and say it was a waste of time; I'd hate to think I've been stabbing myself with a needle every day for nothing.

Once the medical profession came around to the realization that it would take more time than they first predicted to cure MS, the focus switched to trying to stop the progression of the disease. The pharmaceutical companies developed the ABC drugs, but none of these companies can actually verify the efficacy of their product. They have their own test results, but most of the time their results cannot be duplicated by an independent agency. And if the studies are negative they don't even release them.

In spite of the fact that the ABC drugs available are really stopgap measures for the disease, we live in the best time ever right now for the possibility of cures. We may now have reached the first grade in our knowledge of ourselves, our diseases, and our environment. In the next twenty years we'll be seniors in high school; twenty years after that we'll be graduate students. Over the next two decades the science fiction of the Bionic Man will become a reality. We already have many different man-made prosthetics. Computer chips help operate bionic arms. There are high-tech artificial knees, ankles, and hip joints available today. There are electronic devices that keep certain muscles and organs functioning. There are cochlear implants with electrodes attached to the brain, operated by a battery that makes a person hear who has never heard before. There is a mechanical eyeball with its own power source that will send images to the brain. If these exist now, imagine what we'll see twenty years from now. This is what I remind myself when I'm depressed.

Before the ABC drugs, doctors used to recommend that women who had MS get pregnant. Pregnancy seems to suppress MS and in some cases symptoms don't come back for a while. A large percentage of pregnant women with MS find their symptoms dissipate during their second and third trimesters. It may have to do with the thousands of different proteins and hormones that are present inside a pregnant woman's body. One of those proteins is called Alphafetaprotein (AFP), which is present in both mother and child during gestation and is believed to help suppress both the mother's and the fetus's immune system so that they don't attack one another. This protein was researched by a Dr. Abramsky in Israel, supposedly with much success. When he injected it into some MS patients, their symptoms went away completely. The problem is that the only way you can get it is from placentas, and you need a couple of thousand placentas to get enough for one month's treatment for one person. So a company called Merrimack has genetically engineered a goat to produce this protein. It is waiting for approval by the FDA and in several corners of the world it is being looked upon as the silver bullet. It may not cure MS but it just may stop it from progressing any further.

I've been to the company, and as we raise more money I'd like to help fund their research. I believe very strongly in fighting disease the same way I was taught in the military: to go to war with every possible base covered, from the marine corps to the air force to the army and navy. It's the same with MS. The bigger the arsenal in the fight, the better.

I'm not just a contributor or a fund-raiser, of course; I'm also a guinea pig. Every time I go to the Karolinska Institute I have longer and longer MRIs. These are prized by scientists because the longer the magnet spins around, the more refined each slice will be, until it's reached the cellular level. The noise of that whirling steel doughnut is about as loud as a car engine, and it can give you a killer headache. Most people can only take it for forty-five minutes, but I've lain there without moving for as long as eleven hours. I've been through it so many times I've even taught myself to go to sleep in there. Doctors can't believe it!

The researchers were all very excited when I agreed to take an eleven-hour MRI, and it made me excited that they were so excited about what they might get, that my brain could possibly help open another door of insight into this disease. I'm one willing guinea pig. If they want me to lie there for two days, I'll do it. I wish they'd create a facility to collect and study all the MRIs taken of MS patients over the years. Run them through a computer and look for patterns.

You can't put hundreds of thousands, and probably millions, of MRIs together and not be able to come up with something.

I doubt very much that anyone's going to come up with a magic medicine that will cure MS by studying any one aspect of the disease. I've accepted the fact that I may be sticking a needle in my stomach and butt for the rest of my life. But maybe down the line what I'll be sticking in my body will do more than what the current drug I'm taking is doing. Instead of cutting down on my future episodes it will eliminate them, effectively eradicating this disease from me. Then twenty years from now somebody might figure out how to make it in a pill form, and after I'm dead the next generation will get one shot when they're born and they will be completely inoculated against it. There will end up being an immunization for MS, like there is for smallpox and chicken pox.

At Nancy Davis's Race to Erase dinner three years ago, I said I couldn't believe it had been a year since I was diagnosed and the number of people reported with MS didn't change; not only that, but it hadn't changed for twenty years! In that year I'd personally heard from more than 3,000 people who were recently diagnosed, yet the numbers never changed. Inspired, Bradley O'Leary, the president of Associated Television News, who has a family member with MS, immediately asked Zogby International to do a poll to find out from doctors and patients across the country who has MS. The result: 2.76 million people. If those numbers are correct, that would make MS one of the most prevalent diseases in America. Well, nobody wanted to believe it; everyone said the poll must have been flawed. So for the next year and a half I worked very hard to get Gallup to do a poll. The Gallup study of consumers found approximately 960,500 U.S. households have at least one person suffering from MS.

Think about it. If there really are even 1 million people with MS, then the load this is going to have on the U.S. medical and health care system in the next ten years will be formidable. No one is prepared for the number of people who are afflicted. I don't know how the system can handle a million people walking or being wheeled in every month for checkups because of MS. We're going to see a much greater problem than anyone imagined.

The most consistent thing about MS is its inconsistency. The next most consistent thing is that most MS patients are undertreated. And that there are far more people who are suffering from the disease than has been reported. We've come a long way in the last ten years, but we've still got a mountain to climb.

12

Who's That
Black Dude?

My friend Rupert asked me the other day if I was happy.

Am I happy? Not as much as I'd like to be, but I'm working at it. This disease has made me so critical of myself that sometimes I forget to stop and take a look around at the top of that mountain. But I'm aware of that and several times a day I pinch myself to appreciate all that I have.

Because in spite of everything I have said about my struggles with MS, I truly can't look at it as a tragedy. It's not. What I've gone through has opened me up to understanding so much more about myself, about people, about humanity. It's made me value life more. It's made me stop being so judgmental.

I was leaving an amusement park in Cincinnati with my kids last summer when this lady in front of us stopped to rearrange her popcorn, her stuffed-animal prizes, and her handbag, and took what seemed like ten minutes to get going again. We were in a hurry and one of the friends I was with wanted to ask that woman to move out of our way. I held him back. We were not in that big of a hurry. I said, "Ma'am, take your time, and if you want, we'll help you."

Every aspect of my life has changed because of this illness, because I look at life through a different pair of lenses. They might not be rose-colored but they're very sharp. I scrutinize things more and then I try not to judge.

I'm definitely a better person—even just in terms of understanding myself.

I've come a long way from the day that doctor in Utah looked me in the face and told me I had MS. I'll never forget that look. If I could reach back in time and smack him, I would. Because the way he talked to me, the attitude he presented, made me want to kill myself.

If that's the way doctors are diagnosing their patients, with such a lack of empathy or even common courtesy, then is it any wonder that we who are diagnosed with an illness feel so helpless and look upon our futures as hopeless? How many people walk in to see their doctors, find out they have MS, and five months later they're in a wheelchair? Is that because their disease really progressed so quickly or is it because they had some insensitive doctor who said, "Sorry. You have MS. There's nothing we can do about it. You'll just have to take it easier." People go home and lie in their beds at a time when they should be exercising instead, or starting physical therapy. But their doctors told them there was nothing to be done, and so they lie down and live down to someone else's expectation.

I met a woman recently in an airport lounge who walked up to me and said, "I watch your show every day. I have MS and four years ago I was in a wheelchair. I wasn't able to walk, and then you got my butt out of that chair. I felt you were talking to me through the screen."

That's so encouraging. I get crazy when I talk to someone with MS who has no hope. There *is* hope. There are things anyone can do to help himself. We know that messages from the brain often don't reach their intended destinations because of the damage along the central nervous system, so we can work on strengthening the brain, by learning how to play a musical instrument, studying a foreign language, or doing math drills. If we have memory problems, there are mental exercises we can do to help stimulate the areas of the brain where memory occurs. I truly believe the brain has the ability to rewire around a problem area if we stimulate it the right way. People spend more time complaining about what they've lost than seeing what they can do to regain it.

If your job is repetitive, like inputting data on a computer or answering telephones, you have to figure out ways to stimulate your brain. Pick up a crossword puzzle. Read a magazine article and then write down what you've learned until you are able to get all the details down. If you need to sharpen your memory, try tricks like putting things into categories; it helps you memorize and recall information.

We don't challenge people with MS to exercise all their faculties. If you have difficulty balancing, try sitting on a Swiss ball. I met a woman who was in a wheelchair because she had no strength in her legs, no muscle tone. I suggested she do light exercises on a Swiss ball, even if it was a minute a day. I told her she should get her boyfriend to help her out of that wheelchair, hold his hands and try to balance herself on the ball. Then I showed her she could wrap a shoestring around a doorknob and use that along with her legs to keep herself up. And if she could let go of that string and just use her legs to keep from falling, even if only for twenty-five seconds, she could set a goal of twenty-six seconds for the next day. And a second more for each day after that.

If you're in a wheelchair and you can barely lift a cup, well, then, have a physical therapist show you how to reach across your body to pick up that cup. And then have the therapist bring you a one-pound dumbbell to lift. If you can only do one repetition with it on the first day, then try to do two on the second, and three on the third. If you see some improvement, no matter how small, then you will know that you have some control over your disability. And some control is better than no control at all.

If you can only move one finger on your hand, there are exercises you can do with a rubber band to work that finger. At the end of one or two weeks of using a rubber band, that finger may be sufficiently strengthened to help you move the button on your wheelchair better. And if you can move one finger, next week it might be two fingers, the next week three. Those of us who have this disease, at whatever level, are still doing one finger at a time every day. I believe that that is the key to making our quality of life better.

What I'm suggesting should be done under a doctor's or physical therapist's supervision. You just have to seek out a doctor who understands the value of exercise. When your knuckle hurts from that rubber band, as long as it's not causing arthritis or tearing your joints, then I say no pain, no gain. And that goes for anything in life. No gain in relationships unless it's painful emotionally; no gain in anything unless there is a little pain.

It's true for every aspect of this disease. If you say, "No, I can't," then you won't—even though you probably could. We live down to other people's low expectations. If your doctor tells you, "Your disease is so progressive you're going to be bedridden next week," don't get into your bed. Prove him wrong! I won't get into that bed until I can do nothing other than get in that bed. And then when I get in that bed I'm still going to do sit-ups so that when somebody comes and brings me a tray of food I can sit up and eat it. And if I can't sit up and eat, then I'm going to start doing neck-ups. That's what it's about. If not, then the hell with it, you're already dead.

Hopefully you have a loving and caring support system. The people around you need to know they shouldn't accept the words "I can't today." Look at people who have overcome enormous obstacles, like Helen Keller, Beethoven, John Milton or Stephen Hawking. They accomplished so much not only because they believed in themselves, but because someone else believed enough in them to push them. It was undoubtedly painful for them but the results in the end were phenomenal.

I'll never compose a symphony like Beethoven or write verse like Milton or understand the universe like Hawking, but I can relate to the obstacles they each had to overcome. I may be a total wreck half the time, but I'm working every day not to be one.

There are choices. I'm hoping that some of this resonates in the minds of people who don't feel like they have a choice. The reason people don't make the decision to get up and do things is because they think it won't make any difference. Bullshit! People with MS get up out of their wheelchairs every day. We have a choice. We have a choice about everything that happens to us until the day we die. We can make the choice to live a miserable existence or we can make the choice to be happy in spite of everything.

I've been honest about the negatives and the hurts in my life, but I don't want to dwell on them. If I stop for fifteen minutes and contemplate my misery, that misery can overtake me. Instead I choose not to; I choose to live. And even when I'm hurting I try my best to believe that something good can come out of it.

I made a decision the day I got up off that street in Columbus Circle, looking at the car that swerved around me, that even though I have MS, it's not going to have me. Period. They're just six little words: it's not going to have me. But once I said them, I refocused my life. When I get up each morning, I ask myself: What am I going to do today that's worth talking about tomorrow?

I have MS. MS does not have me.

At last year's Race to Erase MS I said in my opening speech that one of the things people with MS need to do is stop lying. And I've been lying. To myself. To others. Hiding my symptoms from friends and family, not telling my doctors how I truly feel, not being open with women who care for me. I make excuses for things that I should not be making excuses for, like tripping or cramping. Maybe I am too critical of myself but I believe that that critical nature in me is also what is helping to keep me motivated and looking to do better. I put up a front that, in some ways, has made me stronger. But it's also why, in the middle of the night when it's dark, I don't sleep.

In my darkness I've wondered why there are diseases like this. And I think maybe it's so man can finally reach his fullest potential. Maybe some of the diseases we get are just our adaptation to nature's curveballs. As we continue to adapt and learn how to treat and boost and cure our immune systems perhaps we won't be so susceptible to disease. Then we will have become genetically superior beings; illnesses that might have destroyed us will have been eradicated. Maybe four, five, six, or seven generations from now we will have evolved to be smarter and stronger and healthier. So is there a reason for disease? I think I'm living with this and fighting this so that if one of my children or grandchildren or great-grandchildren is ever diagnosed with MS they'll be cured.

I expect we will come up with drugs that seem to arrest the disease, but it will take twenty years of being free of symptoms to know if they really work—not enough for me. I know my own chances of being cured are slim to none. My destiny is more likely to be one of slow but continual degradation, but I will continue to do everything in my power to keep it at bay. I truly don't fear death. I fear living with limited capabilities more than I fear dying, so every morning that I wake up and don't stumble out of bed is a good morning.

When Lola Falana was on my show she spoke of how she put her faith in God to help her deal with her MS. I've thought about that, and sometimes I wish I could do the same, but I have a different relationship with God. I pray, almost as a meditation, but my prayers are never for myself and don't speak to anyone in particular.

When I hear about other people's near-death experiences, they often talk about how Jesus or the Virgin Mary came to them. It wasn't Jesus or Mary who came to greet me in the hospital that day I nearly died. And it wasn't an angel or a spirit guide or crossover helper—at least, it wasn't anything like what I might have imagined. It was a shrouded, androgynous *thing* that appeared. It woke me up, made me laugh, brought me back . . . but it didn't give me religion.

I get strength from praying or reading the Bible because there are words in every religion that are very comforting and motivational and inspirational. At the Naval Academy I studied the Koran, the Torah, and a little Eastern religion. Certain aspects of Hinduism really resonated with me, especially the concept that man's net worth is not what he is to himself or his family, but what he is to the world. There are things in our lives that are out of our control. Whether or not we believe in God, it's a good thing to be able to pray and to appeal to some greater power. A sense of spirituality can ease our hearts.

In chapter 7 I made my case for medical marijuana to the president of the United States. If I were given another fifteen minutes with him, I'd make the case for more funding and attention to be paid to MS.

"Mr. President, one of the top priorities that you and this Congress have on your plate is health care. But those who have been advising you about health care haven't taken into account the fact that there may be four or five times as many people with MS as has been reported. The new Gallup and Zogby polls show that there are anywhere from close to a million to 2.7 million people who have MS in this country. If only half of them need additional medical care that is not covered by insurance, we're looking at a minimum of 500,000 to 1.3 million people who are going to tax our health care system to the tune of $100 million to $200 million a year.

"We need to start by changing the status of MS from an orphan disease to a full-fledged disease that the NIH can fund at a level that will lessen its impact on us as a society over the next ten years. We've got to start an all-out war against MS and all other neurological diseases today.

"Bring together some public figures like Christopher Reeve, Michael J. Fox, Muhammad Ali, Richard Pryor, Lola Falana, Nancy Davis, and myself with those private-sector people working on spinal cord damage, Parkinson's, Alzheimer's and MS, and get them to share data, because in the world of neurological disorders and brain atrophy, a breakthrough for any one of them could impel all the others toward a possible cure. *But we need the funding.*

"I realize, Mr. President, that you have a war on terrorism on your hands and that you are shifting funds into the military. But let me point out that the number of MS sufferers in the military is large and continuing to rise. That affects our military readiness, not just in troop strength but financially. And then we have soldiers whose spouses or parents have MS. These soldiers are unable to fully concentrate on their jobs because they're worried about coming home to help their loved ones.

"Mr. President, lead us into this new war, a war against neurological diseases. Demand that the NIH and this nation put their energies and resources into conquering these painful and crippling diseases. Let me and Michael J. Fox and Christopher Reeve be your soldiers. This country declared war against breast cancer and in the last dozen years the results have been remarkable. The survival rate of women with breast cancer continues to rise. Well, unfortunately, the debilitation of sufferers of neurological disorders is going up every day and we need funding to turn the tide."

So much for my extra fifteen minutes with the president. Don't think I'm not trying to get that time. At the same time I'm asking my viewers, and you readers as well, to give what you can, because we all benefit from generosity. If I could have one wish granted it would be for the three people who staff my foundation to lose their jobs because there was no longer a need to raise money to find a cure for MS.

Until then, I'll just keep sticking my face out there, reminding people that all may not be well but that isn't going to stop me. I'm still going to pump iron. I'm still going to race Gooch on a Razor scooter. I'm still going to dance with my daughters. And I'm never going to stop strapping on my snowboard and go gliding down those snow-covered mountains.

Which reminds me . . .

I was snowboarding in Mammoth a year and a half ago when my publicist called and said, "I forgot to tell you, you have to do this photo shoot on Sunday in L.A. for Paramount."

"What kind of photo?"

"Something about the history of Paramount. They want to include you in a picture that will be in *Vanity Fair*."

"I'll pass. It's a great day here and it's going to snow Sunday."

"No, you've got to go."

Man, I didn't even have any decent clothes with me! I had to have my stylist send me some. I was a little irked that nobody had told me anything about this. I hate when that happens. You know, it just throws me.

So I get down to L.A. and drive onto the Paramount lot, right into a swarm of paparazzi. I was thinking, oops, this can't be for me; we should go around the other way. But I got out of the car and reporters started shouting, "Montel, what do you think about this? It's a historic event."

I smiled pleasantly to one and all. "I think it's incredible; it's a wonderful idea." I had no idea what I was talking about! I still didn't know what was going on.

Finally someone asked, "How do you feel about being one of the ninety celebrities coming together for Paramount's ninetieth anniversary?"

Then I looked up, and coming down the hallway were Michael Douglas and Catherine Zeta-Jones. Behind them was Sidney Poitier, and behind him Mickey Rooney, Diane Keaton, Ashley Judd, Harrison Ford, Charlton Heston, Jodie Foster, Sharon Stone . . . I felt like a kid in a candy store. Al Pacino came up to me and said, "Hey, Montel, how you doing?" Al Pacino! Then I said to Tom Cruise, "Did you know we have the same birthday?" And he said, "I know—you, me, and Geraldo!" It tripped me out. Everyone was smiling and friendly, like it was our high school reunion or something. Demi Moore said, "Hi, Montel, how are you?" She was as gorgeous and as sweet as she could be. I must have looked like some kind of slack-jawed fool.

We were told to wait in a holding area, so there I was hanging out with Brendan Fraser when I hear Catherine Zeta-Jones say, "Michael, where's the camera? Gimme the camera. It's Sidney!" And off she goes to ask Sidney Poitier if he'll take a picture with her. A couple of people even asked if they could take a picture with me! At one point I was chillin' with Michael Douglas when Angelina Jolie stopped to say hello. She was two inches from my face and her beauty nearly took my breath away. Morgan Freeman saw that I was starting to hyperventilate. "Breathe, man," he said in that unmistakable voice—no wonder Jim Carrey chose him to play God—"what's the matter?"

I said, "I can't believe this. I'm so starstruck. I don't think I deserve to be here."

"Montel," he said, "you need to stop and just remember something. . . . Take a look around this room. All these people here are actors, but I will bet you a lot of them wish they could do what you do. Because they can't speak, Montel, they can't deal with issues like you do. You belong here. Calm down."

The time came for the picture. There I was surrounded by all these stars: Matthew Perry, Jennifer Beals and Jim Carrey above me; Mike Connors, Kate Mulgrew and Robert Downey Jr. to my left;

David Spade and Anjelica Huston to my right; Jon Voight, Jessica Lange, Helen Hunt, and Samuel L. Jackson below me.

I looked around me and thought about my disease and how blessed I was to have made it there. I was just so grateful that they didn't have to wheel me in. Because this photo was going to last forever. The first one, taken sixty years earlier, was hanging in the lobby of Paramount. This picture would hang right there beside it. A hundred years from now somebody's going to look at it and say, "Who's that black dude in the middle of the picture?"

It's me.

Update

I learned early on in life that nothing fills me up, or builds me up, like a sense of pride. For me, that comes from trying my hardest, being true to myself, and setting and achieving goals. I discovered this about myself as a young boy. It's what sustained me throughout my commission in the navy, and it's a driving force behind my career even now as I enter the fourteenth season of my talk show.

When I was diagnosed with MS in 1999, I felt that I lost so much. The world couldn't see it, but for me, it was the first time I was unsure about my future—as a dad, as an employee, as an employer, as a lover. Before MS, I was sure-footed and knew my path and purpose; with MS I was literally off balance. Before MS, I wanted to share my life with one person, but since my diagnosis that kind of intimacy feels like it comes with too many caveats—too many ways to make myself vulnerable, too many opportunities to be disappointed. For the past five years I hid the fact that fear, not pride, was my greatest motivator.

I'll never forget the woman who made me admit that to myself. To this day, I don't know her name. She's one of the many strangers who come up to me at restaurants, airports and book signings. Usually, people want to thank me for some comfort or encouragement I gave them. Not her. "Montel," she said, "you're doing people with

MS an injustice." The blank look on my face told her I didn't have a clue about what she meant. "I have MS," she explained, "and my husband can't understand why I'm not doing as well as you. You don't look like you're sick. He thinks I shouldn't either."

Whoa! Her husband was comparing her insides to my outsides, and my outsides only told half of my story. If he had any idea about the constant fire in my feet, the depression that has made me want to kill myself, the nights I lay awake in spasms and sweat, maybe then he'd appreciate what his wife was going through. That woman was my wake-up call. She made me realize that I hadn't been completely honest with everyone—heck, I hadn't really been honest with myself.

On January 6, 2004, *Climbing Higher* was published and I sat on the stage of my talk show and, for the first time ever, appeared as a guest on my own show. Emme, who acted as host, helped me unlock the dead bolt I was keeping on my pain, my suffering, essentially on my truth. The tears I unleashed that day were from sadness, from relief and from the fear that comes with baring your soul. But I also cried tears of happiness because I knew that I would no longer be carrying my burden alone. People in the office, my friends, my family, my lovers—everyone would know what I've been holding in for so long.

Was I scared? Hell yes. Was it a risk? Absolutely. I was terrified to say out loud to millions of strangers that I've been depressed and that I've attempted suicide. But depression is prevalent in MS patients and has taken a hold on society in general. I found comfort, unexpectedly, in letters from people who have been there, too, and from passersby hailing me to wish me well on the streets. People do not judge me as weak, as I feared. It is actually the opposite: they see my willingness to speak out as courageous. And rather than isolating me, as my celebrity sometimes does, my brutal honesty about life has brought me closer to my viewers, my loved ones, my friends and colleagues.

There was, however, one thing that conventional wisdom said I shouldn't have shared—that I use medical marijuana. I was positive that this, not my depression, would draw the most attention of anything in the book, but surprisingly, it hasn't. Maybe that's because more than 60 percent of Americans believe in the legalized use of marijuana for medicinal purposes, according to reports published by the Institute of Medicine and in the *Journal of the American Medical Association.*

At one point in our recent history, the federal government did, too. Many people don't know it, but the federal government currently ships medical marijuana to the local pharmacies of seven patients they approved to receive it over fourteen years ago. The first Bush administration closed this program to new applicants in 1991, but the seven surviving patients who entered the program prior to that year are still receiving their monthly allotments of marijuana, which the federal government is growing at the University of Mississippi.

The hypocrisy of the federal government is reprehensible. On the one hand, officials say more research is needed, but on the other hand, they do nothing about the bureaucratic obstacles that continue to slow or even block research on marijuana's therapeutic benefits. One effort to break this logjam—a proposal from the University of Massachusetts to grow marijuana for FDA-approved research—has been stalled at the DEA for three years without action!

This politicking is inconceivable to me, when lives are at stake. Practically everyone knows someone who is suffering from cancer, AIDS, MS, glaucoma, arthritis or migraines, and we deserve some relief from our anguish.

As if living, *and dying*, with chronic illness isn't enough to worry about, imagine having to worry about going to jail because you're using the medicine that your doctors recommend! That's what's happening around the country, where DEA agents are arresting seriously ill patients whose actions are *in compliance with their states' law.* That's why I lobbied Congress in July 2004 in support of the Hinchey-Rohrabacher Amendment, which says that the federal government cannot undermine state laws that authorize the use of medicinal marijuana. If that isn't big government at its worst, I don't know what is!

Opponents of the legalization of medical marijuana argue that it will jeopardize our country's youth, making marijuana more accessible to kids and sending them the wrong message. I am determined to debunk this myth because kids are very important to me. I have four of my own and I started my career by telling kids to stay in school and stay off drugs. My message to them hasn't changed. I am pleased that the California attorney general's office recent California student survey showed that teen use of marijuana has continued to drop markedly since the state's medical marijuana law was passed in 1996. Teens are able to understand the difference between medicine and drug abuse. Why can't adults? I live in New York, and according to a poll by Zogby International, 66 percent of New Yorkers agree that patients should have medically supervised access to marijuana. That support cuts across party lines. As it should! Having the ability to live pain-free and with dignity is a nonpartisan issue. Despite this majority, New York is NOT one of the nine states that allow the use of this natural botanical (California, Colorado, Hawaii, Maryland, Maine, Nevada, Oregon, Vermont and Washington do).

Well, that's just not acceptable to me. Last spring I met with public officials in New York who were considering a measure on behalf of medical marijuana. I looked dozens of legislators in the eyes and let each of them know that I and millions of others are suffering needlessly. I made sure they know that I will not stop talking about this. I will not stop advocating. I will not relent until the day I no longer have to choose between being in pain and being considered a criminal.

I wrote this book as a means to stop and take a look around, and more and more I'm happy with what I see. The shadow of fear that surrounded me when I started this journey has lost its embrace. Now I live in a much more comfortable place, where hope and promise reside. My sense of pride has returned, but today it is inspired less by my accomplishments and more by the candor in my relationships, the quality of time spent with my kids and the fact that I can be who I truly am on my talk show and with all of you. MS is not the death sentence I thought it once was, but it is definitely a big mountain. The key is to continue climbing and to discover ways to enjoy the view.

Appendix
43 Questions Answered:
A Doctors' Roundtable

Throughout the course of this book I have described MS as a blessing. One reason is that I have met so many people I wouldn't have met otherwise, and shared laughter and tears with these complete strangers. I'm not just talking about the thousands of you who have come to a taping of the show or stopped me in the middle of the street or at a book signing to share your story or express words of support. I also mean the doctors who have been my personal coaches and cheerleaders. These are the people who have poked, prodded, scanned and studied me down to the cell. They have answered hundreds of my endless questions and seen me at my most vulnerable. Nevertheless, they continue to lift me up by empowering me with knowledge and by nourishing me with their encouragement. They are a tribute to their profession. These men and women have dedicated their lives to the study of MS, sometimes to the study of just one strand of DNA. They are remarkable people, inside and outside of their labs and offices, and I hold them all in the highest regard. Thanks to them I am much more in touch with myself than I ever was and have learned what a true marvel and miracle the human body is. Thanks to them I not only have an understanding of what is going on in my body, but I also have hope for my future, and all our futures.

When I told each of them that I wanted to present them with some questions about MS, to provide readers with the most up-to-the-minute information, they were eager to share their current research and their predictions for the future. Each doctor brings a unique perspective, born of his or her specialization, to the questions posed below. You will notice that some of their answers contradict one another and, to me, that speaks to the fact that there are still more questions about this disease than there are answers. And it is a poignant reminder that there is still a lot of work that needs to be done. I hope as you read this you will keep in mind what I've been saying all along—that we each have our own version of MS, no two cases are identical. We each must speak with our health care professionals to determine our own best course of action. And we must each take responsibility for our health care.

These doctors are:

Dr. Walter R. Frontera, Chairman, Harvard Medical School Department of Physical Medicine and Rehabilitation; Director of the Muscle Cell Physiology Laboratory at Spaulding Rehabilitation Hospital

Dr. Bernadette Kalman, Director of MS Research at St. Luke's–Roosevelt Hospital Center, Columbia University; Assistant Professor of Neurology, Columbia University

Dr. Adam Kaplin, Chief Psychiatric Consultant to the MS Center at Johns Hopkins University School of Medicine

Dr. Hugo W. Moser, Director, Neurogenetics Research Center, Kennedy Krieger Institute

Dr. Michael J. Olek, Director, UCI Medical Center's Multiple Sclerosis Center

Dr. Tomas Olsson, Director, Department of Molecular Medicine, Karolinska Institute, Stockholm, Sweden

Dr. Howard Weiner, Professor of Neurology, Harvard Medical School; Director MS Center, Brigham and Women's Hospital/Massachusetts General Hospital

A more thorough synopsis of each of these doctors' credentials follows the questions and answers. Please note that not all participants responded to all questions.

DOCTORS' APPROACHES TO AND EXPERIENCES WITH TREATING MS

1. How long have you treated patients who have MS, or how long have you studied the effects of the disease?

Dr. Tomas Olsson: For approximately twenty-three years.

Dr. Hugo W. Moser: Forty years.

Dr. Michael Olek: Ten years.

Dr. Bernadette Kalman: For about fifteen years, which includes both clinical work and basic research.

Dr. Adam Kaplin: My research experience includes having trained under two Nobel Prize winners and doing doctoral and post-doctoral research in the laboratory of Dr. Solomon Snyder, preeminent neuroscientist and founder of the Department of Neuroscience at Johns Hopkins. I have worked in the psychiatry department at Johns Hopkins for the past seven years, where I did my specialty training. I have focused my clinical and research interests on patients with multiple sclerosis and related autoimmune neurologic diseases for the past four years.

Dr. Howard Weiner: Over thirty years. I began my work in 1971.

Dr. Walter Frontera: I have been involved in the rehabilitation of patients with neurological diseases for several years.

2. What is your philosophical approach to treating MS?

Dr. Kalman: It is difficult to describe a general strategy, but considering the current treatment modalities, for most cases an early aggressive use of disease-modifying drugs is probably the most effective approach. However, each patient needs individual evaluation and judgment.

Dr. Weiner: My approach is that of aggressive therapy. I do not believe that we will cure MS by not treating it. Although there are some patients who have benign forms of MS and do well with the disease, the majority of patients over time do not do well. Thus my philosophy is to treat as soon as possible and watch carefully to achieve stabilization in the disease, or if a person is not treated to watch them carefully and to initiate treatment as soon as disease activity occurs.

Dr. Moser: Overall care of all aspects of function, life and disease process.

Dr. Olek: Treat early and aggressively.

Dr. Frontera: From a rehabilitation point of view, my approach is to restore form and function, even though the basic disease cannot be cured yet. We can do many things to enhance the functional capacity and quality of life of the patient with MS using modern rehabilitation techniques.

Dr. Kaplin: This is truly a broad question. To begin, I believe working with patients with MS is necessarily a collaborative endeavor. Helping the patient through the process of understanding and adjusting to their illness, including its unpredictable nature, is a crucial component. Working together to formulate a plan that will employ the best possible therapeutic options while minimizing treatment side effects is crucial. The challenges faced by patients are often multifactorial, arising out of the combined effects of the disease and its treatments on the body and mind. The treatment must therefore be collaborative. The neurologist, physiatrist and physical therapist, urologist, psychiatrist, and internist, to name a few, must communicate with each patient and one another to provide a coherent treatment plan that maximizes the patient's overall well-being.

The goals must be explicitly to focus on the function, quality of life, longevity and comfort of the patient, usually in that order of priorities. Finally, being honest and humble in recognizing the limitations of current understanding and treatment options in MS requires that each physician listen to the individual's coping strategies in addition to focusing on the effects of approved therapeutics.

Dr. Olsson: An overall response to this would be "holistic." The multifaceted aspects of the clinical condition with effects on neurological functions, but also general signs such as fatigue, altered mood and effects on social life (family, work, etc.), necessitates (1) awareness of proper immunomodifying treatment regimens and proper symptomatic treatment of spasticity, pains, bladder disturbances, fatigue, depression, etc., but also (2) ability to provide help with rehabilitation, and (3) social support. This in turn requires an MS team in most cases composed of a neurologist with particular interest in MS, MS nurse, physiotherapist, occupational therapist, social worker and neuropsychologist.

3. How varied are the symptoms of MS?

Dr. Moser: Very.

Dr. Olek: Widely variable.

Dr. Frontera: Variability in symptoms is significant because the lesions can affect many sites in the nervous system.

Dr. Weiner: The symptoms are quite varied and depend on the individual. However there are a common group of symptoms, including trouble with vision, bladder, sensory disturbances, motor function, balance and in some instances pain. Patients may have funny feelings, such as walking on sand. Other parts of MS include fatigue and cognitive changes.

Dr. Olsson: Since the basic disease process with inflammatory focal lesions can hit at almost any site in the CNS (central nervous system), the ensuing focal neurological defects vary considerably between patients. Also the severity of the disease is highly variable with a spectrum from very mild disease over decades to more aggressive courses even shortening life expectancy. In addition, general signs such as fatigue, effects on cognitive function and altered mood varies considerably between persons with MS.

Dr. Kalman: Since MS lesions in the central nervous system randomly hit various anatomical structures, there is a great interindividual variability of the affected structures and the associated symptoms. For example, when inflammation affects the optic nerve(s), the patient has visual loss. In another person the initial lesion may be located in the spinal cord, causing significant loss of motor, sensory and autonomous functions. There are also patients who have significant cognitive problems without much motor impairment.

Dr. Kaplin: Presentations are often as varied as the kinds of people who are affected by the disease. The patients' original constitutional strengths and weaknesses have a dramatic impact on their symptoms, as does the nature and aggressiveness of their clinical progression. The one thing that often will not change throughout the course of the disease is that things will not stop changing, so strategies must be flexible and subject to reappraisal and revision.

4. Do you think that MS may actually represent as many as four different diseases, each with its own pattern of damage, its own cause and its own clinical outlook?

Dr. Olek: Yes.

Dr. Kaplin: I think MS may in fact be the final common pathway of multiple immune processes gone awry. The ultimate expression of this disease is likely influenced by genetic and historical predispositions, environmental insults and the complex interplay between multiple systems within the body. The prognostic significance of describing the course of different patterns of MS is important but needs considerable refinement. At the present time, however, the distinction of classifying MS into different diseases is of limited clinical utility, and often serves only to confuse patients. There is tremendous individual variability even within different patterns of progression in MS, and the clinical outlook cannot be well anticipated at times. This unpredictability should only increase the need for patients and their doctors to be aggressive in trying to minimize long-term disability.

Dr. Kalman: Recent histological studies by Claudia Lucchinetti, Hans Lassmann and colleagues suggested that there may be four types of demyelinating MS lesions based on inflammatory marker profile and myelin staining. These studies were performed using a large number of biopsy and autopsy tissues with acute demyelinating lesions. These analyses are very important since they provided for the first time an objective measure to define subtypes of MS. The four lesion types described by immunohistochemical methods are currently being investigated further. I view inflammatory demyelination as a spectrum of related conditions, and believe that genetic and molecular markers will further refine the classification of MS lesions.

Dr. Moser: There may well be such groups, but there is overlap.

Dr. Weiner: The answer is basically yes, though I wouldn't say there are specifically four diseases. Rather I would say that MS is a syndrome and that there may be different types of MS in different people. The genetic background of each person and environmental exposure causes this. MS in many ways is like the animal EAE model. Animals get different types of diseases depending on the strains, and which myelin protein they are immunized with. I believe one of our challenges in the future is to understand the outlook for individual patients.

Dr. Olsson: The simplest answer to this question is that we do not know. There are, however, some speculations:

First, a group of scientists (Hans Lassmann, Moses Rodriguez, Claudia Lucchinetti and Wolfgang Bruck) have made extensive neuropathological studies on autopsy material and brain biopsies, and claim that there are four different patterns of MS morphologically. It remains to find corresponding laboratory markers to see if this can be studied in living persons with MS, without surgical interventions. There are also certain opponents to this view.

Second, there are strong reasons to believe that there is a genetic predisposition to develop MS. These genes are likely to be normal genes that have been of benefit for survival during evolution, perhaps in the defense against infections; however, as a by-product they give risks for developing MS. There seem to be various genes disposing for the same result (MS-like disease). Thus, one could argue that MS could be regarded as different diseases.

Third, perhaps one should not overinterpret differences in the clinical presentation of MS as a reason to consider MS to be different diseases, because MS in identical twins can have quite different clinical presentations.

WHO DEVELOPS MS?

5. How many people would you estimate have MS in the United States? (Newsweek estimates 400,000. A recent Gallup poll says about 1 million. The Zogby poll says closer to 3 million.)

Dr. Kalman: These different figures may reflect the lack of a comprehensive epidemiological survey, but based on the overall North American prevalence data and the size of the current U.S. population, my estimate would be close to or maybe somewhat higher than the *Newsweek* estimate.

Dr. Olek: 750,000.

Dr. Frontera: I suspect the number may have changed over the last couple of decades due to enhanced diagnosis. Initial estimates may have been too low.

Dr. Moser: I believe in the lower figure.

Dr. Kaplin: We know from autopsy data from the past that MS often goes unnoticed in many patients, and clinical experience has shown that many patients will not seek treatment until their disease proves sufficiently severe. Thus, many cases likely occur at rates that far exceed our current estimates.

Dr. Weiner: I am not qualified to answer this question and am dependent on polls and the new surveys. It does appear that more and more people are being diagnosed with the disease.

Dr. Olsson: Difficult for me as a Swedish resident to have an opinion on this. In our country, which is considered to be a high-risk area for MS, prevalence is close to 0.2 percent, and estimates suggest that 1 out of 500 individuals develops MS during his lifetime. I do not think that too many persons here go undiagnosed.

However, even these numbers are high enough to give the disease an important status also economically for the society. In our population of 9 million people, the yearly cost was recently estimated to be about $600 million. Around 10 percent of this was for drugs, but the major cost is for long-term care of the severely disabled. Less than 1 percent is spent on research on MS.

6. Is MS still considered a "prime of life" disease?

Dr. Olsson: In my understanding of the English, it is. It affects people during the very active parts of their lives.

Dr. Kaplin: Yes.

Dr. Moser: Yes.

Dr. Olek: Yes.

Dr. Kalman: MS can occur in childhood and even in advanced age, but the most common age of onset is in the young adult years.

Dr. Frontera: Yes. It is one of the leading causes of disability in the twenty-to-fifty-year age range, a period of life of significant professional and personal activity.

Dr. Weiner: Yes, MS is a "prime of life" disease. It primarily affects people between the ages of twenty and forty, although there are clearly occasions that it begins after age fifty and it is sometimes seen in children. It is rare for someone over sixty-five to come down with MS at a time when there is an increased incidence of cancer and Alzheimer's disease.

7. Why are people with MS usually diagnosed between the ages of twenty and forty?

Dr. Olek: Unknown.

Dr. Olsson: This is due to the fact that onset of MS is maximal in this age span (max twenty-eight years of age, rarely before age fifteen or after fifty-five).

Dr. Moser: That is when symptoms start most frequently.

Dr. Frontera: The incidence of the disease seems to peak in this age range.

Dr. Weiner: This is when the symptoms begin and damage to the nervous system occurs.

Dr. Kalman: This age of onset may be related to the maturation of the immune system and the completion of myelination or to the nature of interactions between these systems and environmental factors in various stages of development.

Dr. Kaplin: From what we know of neurodegenerative diseases there is often a threshold of brain involvement that must be crossed before symptoms become apparent. Lesions in regions that result in gross neurological deficits tend to present rather quickly. But much of the brain involvement in MS is more subtle, and the disease is likely active for years prior to diagnosis. Unlike some neurodegenerative illnesses that present rather late, such as Parkinson's and Alzheimer's disease, MS is marked by more active inflammation and comes to attention relatively earlier. We therefore may be able to impact this disease more dramatically through earlier intervention to halt progression. Raising public awareness about MS and its common presenting symptoms will likely lead to earlier diagnosis and more successful treatment outcomes.

8. Why do you think people living in certain areas of the world, especially those farther away from the equator, are more susceptible?

Dr. Olek: Unknown.

Dr. Moser: Complex interaction between gene and environment.

Dr. Kaplin: Most likely regional differences are due to environmental exposures, such as infectious agents and perhaps toxic exposures, and genetic predispositions.

Dr. Weiner: This is a complicated question. It probably relates to a number of factors, for example, (1) the genetics of people in different parts of the world; (2) environmental exposure from viruses; and (3) sunlight may play a role, having a beneficial role by affecting immune function.

Dr. Kalman: Both environmental and genetic factors may be responsible for this distribution pattern of MS, but genetics may play a stronger role. Different ethnic groups have different susceptibility to the disease. Scandinavians and their descendants are generally known to have the highest risk, while Lapps living in the northern-most parts of the Scandinavian Peninsula rarely have MS. Gypsies who migrated out of northwest India centuries ago, and settled in various European countries, generally have much lower risk for MS than the Caucasian residents living in the same environments. This varying susceptibility to MS in different ethnic groups suggests a genetic component. Nevertheless, different climatic, geographic and infectious factors may greatly influence the expression of the disease.

Dr. Olsson: One reason is most probably differences in preva-lence of disease predisposing genes in different populations. There is a correlation between the distribution of MS and individuals of Scandinavian origin. There are also possibilities for differences in environmental factors, such as infections, diet and climate. These factors are poorly defined.

9. Is there any truth to the notion that people who work in settings where they are exposed to large groups of individuals, for example teachers and military personnel, are more susceptible to MS?

Dr. Kalman: Some epidemiological studies suggest that while exposure to microbial organisms in early life may shape the immune system in a beneficial way and decrease the risk for autoimmune dis-eases, primary exposures to these organisms in adult life facilitate the development of an autoreactive immune response. Teachers and military personnel are frequently exposed to a great variety of microorganisms in their adult lives through the contact with many children or young soldiers.

Dr. Olek: No.

Dr. Moser: To some extent, but not absolute.

Dr. Kaplin: My opinion, based mostly on clinical experience, is that teachers and nurses get MS more frequently perhaps due to repeated exposures to microbial agents. There is also likely an ascer-tainment bias, because these same groups of patients may be more likely to seek and receive good medical care.

Dr. Olsson: I do not know about any good studies on this matter.

Dr. Weiner: Probably not. Another interesting point is that there is not an increased instance of MS in spouses, suggesting that there is no transmissible viral factor.

WEIGHING IN ON RESEARCH AND ANCILLARY RESOURCES

10. *Until 2000, scientists believed that damage to myelin was permanent. But then testing at the Mayo Clinic showed that giving two human antibodies to mice with the disease caused the myelin to regrow. How far along has this research come and are there possibilities that myelin can regrow in humans affected with MS? Does it mean that MS is reversible?*

Dr. Olek: Possibly.

Dr. Moser: Yes, some regrowth is possible.

Dr. Olsson: In fact I think there were reports already during the 1980s that remyelination regularly took place after myelin damage in MS, by oligodendrocyte precursors maturing into oligodendrocytes. This does not always happen and with time scar tissue develops and nerve fibers are not remyelinated. The nude nerve fibers are then easy victims for damage with permanent neurological defects as outcome. This is an important area for research. Several questions are to be solved. Why does remyelination not always take place? Are there inhibiting factors that can be neutralized? From our lab we know that endogenous stem cells mature into oligodendrocytes after demyelination in rodents. Is the stem cell pool exhausted with time and if so can it be replenished?

At early stages, MS should be reversible. However, in longstanding cases, where a lot of nerve fiber damage has occurred, defects are likely to be permanent.

Dr. Kaplin: Numerous studies have supported the notion that there are varying degrees of regeneration, most often incomplete, seen in lesions of MS patients. This creates the potential to maximize the regeneration process and remove impediments to its completion. In order to do this, not only the inhibitory CNS processes that limit regeneration must be considered, but also the ongoing inflammation and gliosis (or brain "scarring") must be ameliorated. A growing appreciation of the axonal injury that takes place in MS suggests that improving remyelination is only one of several necessary steps that must be undertaken to address the devastating consequences of this disease.

Dr. Weiner: It is possible to help myelin regrow and there are different ways in which it can happen. The body naturally repairs itself and this occurs when there is less of an immune attack on the nervous system in MS. Thus, MS is reversible by its own healing; however once permanent scar formation occurs, it probably cannot heal.

Dr. Kalman: Most scientists believe that there is even a physiological regeneration of myelin (at least to some degrees), which may be further enhanced by natural antibodies. Early during the pathological process of MS, when axons and neurons are still preserved, a remyelination promoting strategy may be beneficial and is not far from the clinical practice. However, the major pathological correlate of disability is the neuronal and axonal degeneration developing secondary to inflammation and leading to progressive atrophy of the spinal cord and brain. Once axonal loss developed, a remyelination promoting strategy could provide very limited or no benefit. For proper conduction of an electric signal from a cortical neuron to a spinal mononeuron we need myelinated axons (processes of nerve cells wrapped with the insulating myelin). Demyelinated axons may still slowly conduct signals, but once axons are transected or degenerated, no signal transfer can be expected in that pathway. Thus, we need to develop strategies to decrease inflammation and to prevent the development of the associated neurodegeneration in order to prevent the development of progressive disability.

11. Are you familiar with the National MS Society's Lesion Project? If so, what is your opinion of it? (According to the NMSS, the MS Lesion Project is a five-year, $1.8 million project. The investigators are analyzing MS lesions in brain tissues from biopsies and autopsies to identify the types of immune cells and other immune factors involved with tissue destruction. The investigators are also *examining clinical characteristics of the individuals from whom these tissues were taken, including clinical symptoms and stages of disease, response to therapy, magnetic resonance images, and immune characteristics of blood samples.)*

Dr. Kalman: It is a very important project. We need markers to better describe subtypes of lesions, correlate the lesions with clinical forms of the disease and define treatment strategies according to the biological behavior of the subtypes of the disease.

Dr. Olek: Yes, it is a wonderful program.

Dr. Olsson: I am not familiar with the lesion project.

Dr. Kaplin: I am not familiar with this project.

Dr. Moser: Neither am I.

Dr. Weiner: Nor I.

12. Is there anything you would like to see the government do—or not do (in terms of accessibility of treatment and ancillary resources, and research for a cure)?

Dr. Olek: More research funds.

Dr. Olsson: As to care, our patients do not have enough access to periods of rehabilitation. As to research, I would like to see much more money spent on research that could lead to better therapy. As discussed above, the proportion spent on research compared to the total cost to society is minute.

Dr. Weiner: Funding of basic research is very important, as is funding of clinical trials. The central question in my mind is whether a network of centers of excellence for the study of MS should be set up by the government/MS Society/private foundations, although this is very expensive and a very politically charged topic.

Dr. Kalman: NIH and other governmental/nongovernmental funding agencies are becoming increasingly aware of the enormous resources required for a successful research project on MS. Therefore, efforts have been made to integrate the intellectual, patient, laboratory and computer resources, and coordinate the individual projects.

Dr. Kaplin: I would like to see the government willing to support both conventional approaches as well as novel ideas in MS research, free from the politics and rhetoric that has proven itself so divisive, misleading and counterproductive in recent years. I would like to see funds also allocated to work that is collaborative, bringing together individuals from different disciplines to provide a cross-fertilization of ideas and approaches.

Dr. Frontera: More services should be available, and maybe more important we have to make sure that patients have access to excellent care, including rehabilitation services. The area of rehabilitation is many times undervalued by payers.

FOOD, DIET AND SUPPLEMENTS IN THE MANAGEMENT OF MS

13. How important is diet in the management of MS?

Dr. Olek: Not important.

Dr. Moser: Not proven.

Dr. Olsson: My guess is that it is not important. However, there is a lack of studies in this area, perhaps due to the fact that such studies are difficult to perform. Furthermore, there are some theoretical reasons based on animal experimentation suggesting that diet could be important. For example, oral tolerance and certain proteins in milk products are similar to myelin proteins, which could have implications for immunological tolerance. Whether milk and/or for example meat consumption would be good or bad for MS is impossible to say with the data available. Thus, I feel that at the present time one cannot give any precise recommendation to a person with MS regarding their diet.

Dr. Weiner: A healthy diet is important. I refrain from telling people that a specific diet will change the course of MS.

Dr. Kalman: I am not aware of any scientifically established diet that would alter the natural history of the disease. However, there are several MS-associated conditions that can be significantly improved with certain dietary measures. For example, patients with

MS often have low vitamin B_{12} levels, which can be tested and easily corrected. The disability-related inactivity and some MS medications (e.g., corticosteroids) cause demineralization of bones. Therefore, vitamin D and calcium replacement can be beneficial for many patients. Constipation is a common symptom of the involvement of the autonomous nervous system. A high-fiber diet can significantly improve this common complaint. Generally, I would recommend to all patients to take a well-balanced diet rich in proteins, fibers, essential amino acids, vitamins and minerals. For any special condition, I would recommend consulting with the specialist who takes care of the patient.

Dr. Kaplin: I do not believe there is much scientific evidence offering guidance for dietary or supplemental approaches to managing MS. I also worry about the lack of standardization, quality control and regulation that exists in the dietary supplement industry. Having said that, I think this is an important area for further research. I also believe that in moderation patients who are so motivated can benefit from experimenting themselves with what works best, especially if it gives them increased control over how they manage and approach their illness.

14. Would you recommend a low-fat diet?

Dr. Kalman: Not for MS. But an MS patient may also have high serum lipids and cholesterol, which need dietary restrictions.

Dr. Weiner: In terms of a low-fat diet, I don't specifically recommend it.

Dr. Olek: Yes, for general health.

Dr. Olsson: Perhaps in general, but not because of MS.

Dr. Moser: No.

15. There are those who advocate a diet high in essential fatty acids, using polyunsaturated fats. What is the reasoning behind this and what do you think?

Dr. Kalman: The reasoning is related to the high lipid and polyunsaturated fatty acid content of myelin. Although such a diet would not hurt, not much benefit regarding the course of the disease and development of progressive disability can be expected from it.

Dr. Weiner: There is logic to having a diet high in essential fatty acids and polyunsaturated fats. The reasoning relates to the immune system, although it hasn't been proven.

Dr. Olek: It is not specific to MS patients.

Dr. Moser: Omega-3 fatty acids reduce immune response.

16. *Do food sensitivities and other environmental allergies play a role in the disease?*

Dr. Moser: No.

Dr. Olek: No.

Dr. Weiner: I do not believe that food sensitivities or environmental allergies play a major role.

Dr. Kalman: Some investigators suggested the involvement of milk proteins, amalgam (filling of the tooth) and other environmental allergies in the development of MS, but there is not enough scientific evidence to confirm these hypotheses.

Dr. Olsson: I am not well informed on this topic, and I think there is a lack of good studies. There have been reports suggesting that allergic diseases such as asthma may recruit an immune response that could be partly protective in MS, but this needs to be confirmed.

17. *Would you recommend that MS patients get tested for food allergies?*

Dr. Olek: Yes.

Dr. Weiner: No.

Dr. Moser: No.

Dr. Olsson: I do not know any sound basis for such testing in MS.

Dr. Kalman: Most people are aware of their food allergy. Avoiding an unnecessary exposure to the offending food may be wise not only for preventing, for example, an unpleasant skin reaction, but also for preventing the potential immune activation and a possible associated worsening of MS symptoms.

18. Is it advisable to eliminate milk products, caffeine, sugar, and yeast?

Dr. Weiner: No.

Dr. Olsson: Not with the present knowledge. In the field of MS, you find enthusiastic proponents of a whole range of different regimens, in most cases unproven, and they may impinge on the quality of life for the person affected with MS. Sometimes also very expensive nonproven treatments are offered, hitting the person economically.

Dr. Kalman: There is not enough scientific evidence to make such a recommendation for MS.

Dr. Moser: No.

Dr. Olek: No.

19. Runners drink mineral water to reduce lactic acid in their muscles. Can mineral water be used to reduce cramping in MS patients? What about calcium?

Dr. Olek: No.

Dr. Moser: No.

Dr. Weiner: The cramping in MS relates to problems in the spinal cord, not to the muscles. But if mineral water helps a person's symptoms, it can be tried.

Dr. Kalman: The causes of exercise-related and MS-related muscle cramps are different. There are several routinely used muscle relaxants, which can diminish spasms and cramping in MS.

Dr. Olsson: I do not think mineral water or calcium would alter the cramps in persons with MS. The reasons are to be found in the spinal cord and are due to lack of inhibitory nerve impulses on motor neurons in the spinal cord.

Dr. Frontera: Runners drink water and drinks with low content of minerals and carbohydrates to replace fluids and salt lost in sweating during the exercise and to provide some fuel for the active muscles. MS patients can do the same thing, especially in relation to physical activity. Replacing fluids and salt can help regulate body temperature better, which is important for MS patients since high temperatures may exacerbate symptoms. Better fluid and mineral balance can help prevent one type of muscle cramps but not all of them. Mineral water may be okay but should not be recommended as a solution to all muscle symptoms.

SIDE EFFECTS AND RELATED SYNDROMES

20. Is a form of herpes associated with all MS patients—and if so, what is the significance?

Dr. Moser: Not proven.

Dr. Olek: No.

Dr. Weiner: Not to my knowledge.

Dr. Kaplin: There is provocative evidence that although not conclusive suggests some infectious agents such as herpes viruses may trigger the immune system to become aggressive toward a patient's own CNS through a process of molecular mimicry. In this theoretical scenario, the virus tries to evade detection by appearing similar to proteins found to be naturally occurring in the CNS. If the virus is detected and the immune response is stimulated, the similar proteins of the CNS may inadvertently be identified as foreign and damage may ensue.

Dr. Olsson: Infections are likely to take part in triggering of MS relapses and there is a series of possible mechanisms how this could take place. However, many MS researchers, including myself, would argue that a very broad spectrum of infectious agents could do this. Studies in adopted children suggest that the social microenvironment has no role—arguing strongly against "specific" MS viruses.

Dr. Kalman: Epidemiological and molecular studies implicate some DNA viruses (herpes simplex virus or HSV 6 and 8 and EBV) in MS. However, it is not clear if these viruses are causative agents or merely show associations with the disease secondary to the underlying immune abnormalities.

21. Is there a higher incidence of stroke among MS patients?

Dr. Olek: Unknown.

Dr. Weiner: I am not aware that stroke is higher in MS patients.

Dr. Moser: I do not believe it is.

Dr. Kalman: MS is associated with other immune conditions (e.g., lupus erythematosus), which can cause vasculopathy or involve antibody production (e.g., antiphospholipid antibodies) associated with hemodynamic problems. The lack of physical activity due to disability may also increase the risk for vascular complications in some individuals.

Dr. Kaplin: Inflammation within the CNS is ultimately toxic in significant amounts, and produces a cascade of responses that can have diverse effects on the entire functioning of the constituents of the brain and spinal cord.

Dr. Olsson: I must confess that I was unaware of studies on this matter. If it is so, it is very interesting. One could consider mechanisms like inflammation. Atherosclerosis is nowadays considered in part to be an inflammatory disease. There could be similar risk predisposing genes for this and MS. One could consider inflammation in the CNS as in MS disposing for vessel occlusions and brain infarcts. These are pure speculations from my side.

22. *MS is considered a neurological disease, but could it also be a vascular disease as well as a disease of the immune system? A metabolic disorder? A genetic disorder?*

Dr. Olek: Yes.

Dr. Olsson: The answer to this question is yes. Early in disease evolution there is inflammation around small vessels in the CNS. Animal studies strongly suggest that the immune system is involved. One can get very MS-like diseases in rodents by immunizing them with myelin components, raising an autoimmune response, in turn giving inflammation in the CNS. Metabolism is more difficult. However, we have reasons to believe that "nervous system metabolic" differences between individuals due to subtle genetic differences may decide how vulnerable the nervous system would be to inflammatory damage. Thus the same degree of inflammation would then give completely different outcomes with regard to neurological defects in different individuals. There is a need for further research on this topic.

As discussed above one could argue that MS is a genetic disease with concordance rates in identical twins of about 30 percent, compared to 2 percent in fraternal twins. There are probably ten to fifty normal genes that modestly affect the risk of getting MS. These will be important to find since they will help identify targets for new therapies.

Dr. Moser: Neurology, immune, genetic, infectious.

Dr. Frontera: Yes, a dysfunctional immune system may contribute to the disease. A genetic basis for the disease has also been suggested.

Dr. Kaplin: MS is undoubtedly a disease that involves the dysregulation of the immune system leading to neurologic injury. Because the brain controls the vital manifestations of our thoughts, emotions and behavior, and these processes have proven exquisitely sensitive to the inflammatory changes that take place in this disease, MS is also a neuropsychiatric disease. With depression occurring in up to 60 percent of patients with MS, and cognitive impairment in up to 50 percent of patients, these manifestations are as common as they are devastating. And these sequelae should not be considered separate illnesses, any more than bladder or sexual dysfunction, but rather the direct consequences of brain involvement from the MS itself. A growing body of research has begun to suggest that not only does MS involve immune-mediated depression, but depression when untreated can result in worsening immune dysregulation and brain injury. Suicide, which largely results from depression, is the third leading cause of death in MS, and usually occurs in relatively young individuals without considerable disability. Of all the consequences of MS, depression is the most treatable when diagnosed, but often goes unrecognized.

Dr. Weiner: I do not believe that there is evidence for MS to be a vascular disease. Some parts of it may be genetic, although this doesn't identify the cause. MS is not metabolic. Rare forms of MS or primary progressive MS may not be immune mediated.

Dr. Kalman: Much evidence suggests a genetic determination of susceptibility to MS. In contrast, we do not believe that the primary underlying pathology of lesion development involves metabolic or vascular abnormalities. Nevertheless, secondary to inflammation we can detect focal metabolic abnormalities in plaques or vascular lesions in some forms of inflammatory demyelination (e.g., Devic's disease).

23. If MS research involves neurology, virology, immunology, epidemiology, and genetics, why hasn't there been a merging of scientific thought to bring all these fields together?

Dr. Frontera: Good question. There must be an effort to enhance the collaboration of scientists with different backgrounds and expertise. This is of special importance when studying conditions that are multisystemic.

Dr. Moser: It exists to a considerable extent.

Dr. Kalman: There has been much effort to integrate observations from various fields. Data from epidemiological studies prompted researchers to start studying molecular genetics. Immunological and virological data are also interrelated. Among candidate genes of MS, we also investigate immune regulatory molecules and mediators of an antiviral response. Thus the observations are neither independent nor obtained independently. However, many of the data need further investigations and clarifications in order to contribute to a solid, integrated view of MS.

Dr. Olsson: I think that there already has been a merging. And more cross-disciplinary scientific work is to be expected.

Dr. Weiner: There indeed has been a merging of all of these areas and a fallacy in some people's thinking is that no one is looking or trying to integrate the different factors that relate to MS. Indeed, most investigators apply all of these factors toward understanding the disease and developing therapies. The National Library of Medicine provides real-time data on current MS research.

Dr. Kaplin: As people learn more and more about less and less, the process of specialization occurs and one of the consequences of this is balkanization of related disciplines. Collaboration is as important on the scientific and research level for MS as it is for the clinical care of those afflicted with this disease. The role of treating physicians should not be underestimated for research, because they recognize the interrelationships between the clinical implications of these various scientific disciplines. Listening to patients and their advocates is also crucial to ensure the research agenda is consistent with their clinical needs and to focus work on areas that result in the greatest suffering.

A model for multidisciplinary research at its best can be learned from studies of MS in African-American populations. This epidemiological research, which showed that MS was roughly half as common in African-Americans but frequently more aggressive in this population, has led to important and exciting genetic research that is beginning to identify candidate genes involved in MS pathogenesis. Similarly, research into the ways in which cytokines may mediate both depression and cognitive impairment has begun to shed light on some of the basic mechanisms by which the immune system can lead to CNS dysfunction.

MEDICATIONS AND THERAPIES

24. What types of medications do you recommend to relieve the various symptoms of MS (fatigue, spasms, pain, etc.)?

Dr. Olsson: Fatigue: in milder cases instructions to rest at certain intervals and adaptation of work, etc.; in more severe cases modafinil can be tried and in a few instances even amphetamines.

Spasms: in most cases baclofen in individualized doses.

Pain: depending on type of pain, amitriptyline, carbamazepine or gabapentin (Neurontin).

Depressions are treated in standard ways with counseling and appropriate drugs.

Dr. Kalman: There are excellent symptomatic medications available to control fatigue, spasms and pain. Each case, however, requires individual evaluation and selection from the numerous pharmaceutical options.

Dr. Weiner: There are several medicines for fatigue, spasms, and pain. These are well known and written about in many sources.

Dr. Olek: Amantidine, Provigil, Cylert, Klonopin, Tegretol, baclofen, Zanaflex, Detrol, etc.

Dr. Moser: Baclofen for antispasticity.

Dr. Kaplin: All medications are toxins, some of which possess beneficial side effects from which they derive their clinical utility. Recognizing the negative side effects that can be caused by medications, such as fatigue by baclofen or cognitive impairment by sedatives, can prevent poor clinical outcomes.

What is very common in MS, and all too often missed, is depression. Depression alone often accounts for the majority of fatigue in MS patients. Similarly, depression often leads to poor sleep. The combination of depression and poor sleep dramatically lowers the pain threshold, making a bearable degree of discomfort immobilizing and intractable. It is not uncommon to see depressed patients treated with stimulating medications to combat fatigue during the day and sedatives to help combat the insomnia caused by stimulant use. With antidepressant treatment and resolution of the depression, both the fatigue and insomnia are often relieved. If, after having ruled out other causes, the symptoms are found to result primarily from the MS directly, symptomatic treatment is indicated. Modafinil (Provigil) and amantadine often assist with fatigue. Spasms can be treated with baclofen, tizanidine (Zanaflex), diazepam (Valium) or tiagabine (Gabatril). Neuropathic pain is assisted by gabapentin (Neurontin), antiepileptic medication and tricyclic antidepressants.

25. Would you recommend vitamin and mineral supplements, and if so, which ones?

Dr. Moser: No.

Dr. Olek: Yes—multivitamin.

Dr. Olsson: Not regularly. We test for vitamin B_{12} and if low, persons get a prescription for this vitamin. Many persons with MS take vitamins, and if in low or moderate doses I do not interfere with this. One should know that certain vitamins can be neurotoxic at high doses.

Dr. Kaplin: I do not believe there is much scientific evidence offering guidance for dietary or supplemental approaches to managing MS. I think it an important area for further research. I also believe that in moderation patients who are so motivated can benefit from experimenting themselves with what works best for them, especially if it gives them increased control over how they manage and approach their illness.

Dr. Frontera: This depends partly on the completeness of the diet and the level of physical activity. A nutritional analysis would be a good start. Higher levels of physical activity could require a general multivitamin/mineral supplement.

Dr. Kalman: As mentioned above, vitamin B_{12} and D, calcium and other mineral supplementation may be necessary for specific causes (e.g., B_{12} deficiency, drug-induced osteoporosis, etc.). Otherwise, a general rule of thumb is that these supplements most likely do not alter the disease course, and their excessive intake may even cause complications. In regards to general well-being, getting vitamins and minerals from food seems to be the most effective.

Dr. Weiner: I do not recommend specific vitamins, although if people want to take a vitamin, I advise a multivitamin, vitamin E and vitamin C.

26. *Would you recommend doing regular exercise, physical therapy and/or yoga?*

Dr. Olek: Yes.

Dr. Moser: Yes.

Dr. Weiner: I think exercise is extremely important. Swimming is important. It is good for the mental status and for the nervous system.

Dr. Kaplin: Regular exercise is good for general health maintenance, and even more important in MS. Exercise with physical therapy cannot only maximize functional independence—it probably stimulates repair of the damage to the CNS and may enhance functional recovery through excitation of neighboring pathways in the brain.

Dr. Frontera: All of them can be useful at different points in time. If the disease has resulted in significant muscle weakness, loss of joint range of motion, soft tissue injuries and contractures, physical therapy may be indicated. Clearly, when more serious complications such as spasticity and neurogenic bladder occur, and performance of activities of daily living becomes impaired, it may be necessary to receive inpatient physical and occupational therapy and rehabilitation services.

When the disease is more stable, a general conditioning program is indicated, including exercises to maintain or increase flexibility, muscle strength, and cardiovascular endurance. Yoga may be helpful for relaxation and flexibility training.

Dr. Kalman: Physical therapy and regular exercise can be both physically and emotionally very beneficial, and therefore are very important elements of our therapeutical armamentarium. Inactive muscles develop atrophy over time, which can further increase the motor disability. Physical activity can prevent atrophy, improve spasms and also facilitate the best functional utilization of the residual motor skills. Yoga can also be rewarding both physically and cognitively. Many people believe that our mind (at least to some degree) can control our body (including the activity of our immune system and other basic mechanisms contributing to MS). However, all these measures can only be supplementary to the available medical therapies.

Dr. Olsson: I recommend physical exercise to all persons with MS, in many cases under the guidance of a physiotherapist. There are good studies showing that this is of benefit for the patients, probably through giving compensating reserve capacity.

27. What do you think about evening primrose oil and fish oils?

Dr. Olek: Okay to use.

Dr. Weiner: I don't think there has been a clear benefit.

Dr. Olsson: No idea.

28. Is there an established connection between mercury and MS? If so, should people with mercury dental fillings have them replaced— just to be on the safe side?

Dr. Olek: No, no.

Dr. Olsson: In my mind there is no evidence for a connection to MS. Dental-filling replacement will just cause some pain and cost money. If a person is obsessed with this, I usually do not argue against replacement.

Dr. Weiner: No. There is no connection and people should not have their fillings replaced.

Dr. Kalman: There is not enough solid evidence to support this notion.

Dr. Moser: No.

Dr. Kaplin: No credible evidence currently is available linking MS and mercury, although this does not disprove a potential connection. Minimizing mercury exposure in moderation is probably reasonable for those individuals worried about this possibility. In the absence of data to support this practice, removal of dental fillings is a good idea primarily for dentists who stand to gain considerably from this expensive procedure.

DECODING MS AND ARRESTING ITS SYMPTOMS

29. Is the attempt to alter the course of the disease through the treatment of the immune system the best hope for the future?

Dr. Moser: Yes.

Dr. Olek: Yes.

Dr. Weiner: Yes, I believe that is the best hope for the future. The other best hope is understanding the degenerative processes that occur in the nervous system.

Dr. Frontera: It is an important attempt but we should not exclude other potential therapeutic avenues.

Dr. Kaplin: At present, there are three general approaches, all of which deserve considerable research and support. The neuroimmunologic approach to treat the effects of the immune system on the CNS is one. Another is the neuroprotective approach, which seeks to preserve and protect the neuronal functioning despite recent or ongoing inflammation. Finally, the neurorestorative approach seeks to find ways, such as stem cells, to repair injured neurons and rewire severed signaling pathways in the CNS.

Dr. Kalman: Immune modulation with interferon beta-1a (Avonex, Rebif) and interferon beta-1b (Betaseron, Betaferon) preparations and with glatiramer acetate (Copaxone) is certainly an important element of our therapeutical armamentarium, particularly in relapsing-remitting (RR) MS. These agents act through complex mechanisms.

There are also new candidate drugs that target single molecules and seem to have significant in vivo immune regulatory effects. Since the activity of the immune system can be altered through different molecular pathways, a combination of immune-modulatory drugs with different molecular mechanisms may result in synergistic effects. This combination strategy merits further investigations and clinical studies. In addition, prevention of neurodegeneration/neuroprotection may be equally or even more important than a mere immune manipulation, particularly in progressive forms of MS. We hope that in the future a combined use of immune-modulatory and neuroprotective medications may be more potent than the currently used immune drugs alone.

Dr. Olsson: As MS at least in its early stages most likely is an immune-mediated disease, it is likely that interference in this system is a way to go. One would like these treatments to be as selective for MS as possible, since we continuously need our immune system in the defense against infections. Here is the challenge.

30. Can you comment on such treatments as immunosuppressants, immune system modifiers, and immune system desensitization?

Dr. Weiner: These drugs have shown to help MS, especially in inflammatory stages. The development of more specific, less toxic medicines that can be given early in the disease I believe will ultimately lead to our controlling MS better.

Dr. Kalman: Immune modulators (interferon beta-1a, interferon beta-1b, glatiramer acetate) have been approved by the FDA because they have some proven benefits in RR-MS. For certain patients, with very active disease and insufficient response to the standard immune-modulatory agents, administration of immunosuppressive medications may be necessary. Immunosuppressive medications are also empirically given to patients with progressive forms of the disease, but often with relatively small benefit. Since not a single antigen can be made responsible for inducing the disease, immune desensitization does not seem to be a very practical and promising approach at this point.

Dr. Olek: Immunosuppressants are the most potent.

Dr. Olsson: Immunosuppressants are not so attractive since they broadly suppress the immune system needed against infections. However, in certain cases of MS with an aggressive course, mitoxantrone has proven useful.

31. What about some of the drugs like azathioprine (Imuran)? Cyclosporine (Sandimmune)? Chlorambucil (Leukeran)? Cyclophosphamide (Cytoxan)? Mitoxantrone (Novantrone)?

Dr. Olek: Very useful.

Dr. Kaplin: For short-term use in patients with aggressive cases until better treatments become available, these types of treatments can have significantly beneficial results in slowing disease progression. Having said that, all of these treatments suffer from being nonspecific and too toxic to consider them optimal. One of the pressing therapeutic needs in MS is to develop less toxic and more specific treatment alternatives.

Dr. Olsson: Data are dubious for most of these, apart from mitoxantrone, where there are clearly benefits for persons with an aggressive course of MS.

Dr. Weiner: Of all the drugs listed we found that cyclophosphamide is the most effective drug for active inflammatory disease followed by mitoxantrone. Cyclosporine is no longer used as is not chlorambucil. Imuran has a mild to moderate effect in MS.

Dr. Kalman: Mitoxantrone is approved for secondary progressive and worsening RR-MS in patients poorly responding to the standard immune-modulatory treatments.

Early aggressive use of cyclophosphamide has been recently tested and may be promising in RR-MS. Azathioprine, an old and inexpensive drug, may also provide benefit in selected patients. The other immunosuppressive drugs are less commonly used, and no sufficient data are available from trials to make a definitive statement about their indications.

Dr. Moser: Depends upon results of controlled trials.

32. *Please comment specifically on the use of chemotherapy drugs in the treatment of MS.*

Dr. Weiner: Chemotherapy drugs, especially cyclophosphamide and mitoxantrone, can help patients with very active inflammatory disease that has not responded to current disease modifiers. If used judicially, it can make a major difference. The chemotherapies point the way to developing new drugs with strong actions.

Dr. Kalman: Chemotherapy (or immunosuppressive therapy) may be beneficial in some patients with highly active inflammatory response, which cannot be sufficiently controlled by the standard approved immune modulatory drugs. However, chemotherapeutical agents usually have severe side-effect profiles, significant associated morbidity and even mortality. Therefore, a careful individual evaluation of the cost and benefit ratio is necessary for each candidate patient considered for such therapy.

Dr. Moser: Not recommended until there are more data.

Dr. Olsson: Not so attractive in view of side effects, but sometimes unavoidable.

Dr. Olek: I use them extensively.

33. *If MS is the result of an abnormality in the blood's lymphocytes, some scientists believe that a transfer of lymphocytes from a healthy, compatible donor should correct the problem. What do you think of this transfer factor?*

Dr. Olek: Worth trying.

Dr. Moser: Needs further study.

Dr. Kalman: This "lymphocyte transfer" was carried out in the form of lymphocytapheresis many years ago, but with unimpressive results. More recently, bone marrow transplantation was tried. This latter procedure requires a bone marrow donor closely matched for the human leukocyte antigens (HLA) with the recipient; immune suppression of the recipient; extensive hospitalization; posttransplant medications and close follow-up. Empirical evidence suggests that the benefit of bone marrow transplantation is modest in MS, the associated mortality rate is unacceptable, and the morbidity is also much higher than with standard medications.

Nevertheless, there might be carefully selected individual cases when this heroic intervention may need to be considered.

Dr. Olsson: Since such a transfer would require genetic identity between donor and recipient, it is not a realistic approach.

Dr. Kaplin: Donor compatibility (i.e., achieving a perfect match) is difficult in this scenario. Moreover, blood cells would die and need to be replenished through repeated transfers, and this treatment would not likely address the established lesions in the brain.

Dr. Weiner: You cannot transfer lymphocytes from one person to the other, as one cannot cross histocompatability barriers. So this is not a viable option.

34. Do you think we will find answers to what is really wrong with the immune system with MS patients?

Dr. Olek: Yes.

Dr. Moser: No.

Dr. Weiner: Yes. I think we already have an insight into what is wrong in the immune system. As more is learned about the immune system, this knowledge will grow.

Dr. Kaplin: We will find answers to what is wrong with the immune system in MS patients and my hope is that gains in this area will come swiftly and guide rational therapeutics. Better understanding of what causes immune tolerance to break down in MS will undoubtedly benefit all patients with autoimmune diseases, as research on these diseases will likely benefit patients with MS.

Dr. Olsson: I personally believe that further translational research in rodent models and in clinical materials combining genetics and immunology will unravel the disease mechanisms.

Dr. Kalman: Ten years ago, I did not really hope that there would be a molecular definition of MS in my lifetime. After witnessing the outcome of the Human Genome Project and the results of the Decade of the Brain, I am quite optimistic regarding the understanding and treatment of MS.

35. What foreign body, or antigen, is the immune system responding to?

Dr. Olek: Unknown.

Dr. Weiner: It appears the immune system is reacting to components of myelin in the central nervous system. This reaction is most likely triggered by a virus or perhaps a limited infection of the brain.

Dr. Kalman: Probably a few antigens are recognized in the early stage of the disease, but the specificity of antigen recognition by T lymphocytes becomes broader and broader through the mechanism of epitope spreading during the course of the disease. Immune recognition of myelin-related antigens (particularly myelin basic protein, myelin oligodendrocyte glycoprotein, proteolipid lipoprotein) has been most extensively studied. Cross-recognition of some myelin protein epitopes and viral proteins by T lymphocytes has been suggested as a potential mechanism of autoimmunity. However, we don't know if the myelin-related antigens recognized by T cells are involved in the induction of the disease or are released and recognized because of the ongoing tissue damage. It is also possible that the virus-specific immune response in MS results from an aspecific activation of memory cells.

Dr. Olsson: Since very MS-like diseases can be induced in rodent models with myelin autoantigen they are likely to be autoantigens of relevance also in human MS. My personal favorite is myelin oligodendrocyte glycoprotein (MOG). It may also be that several CNS proteins simultaneously or at different phases are relevant as target autoantigens.

Dr. Moser: Viral antigen that resembles myelin components.

Dr. Kaplin: This may be different for different people with MS. MS may be the final common pathway of multiple types of losses of immune tolerance in the CNS.

36. *Certain studies indicated that autoimmune diseases might be prevented if wayward T cells could be wiped out before symptoms ever appear. What do you think?*

Dr. Olek: Yes.

Dr. Olsson: This is a futuristic hope that might be possible, and I would not exclude it.

Dr. Moser: Needs further study.

Dr. Kaplin: At present we do not have specific markers for autoimmune T cells that likely mediate much of the errant immune response. This may be a valuable line of research for the future.

Dr. Weiner: It is probably impossible to wipe out wayward T cells because the T cells that can cause MS are part of the normal repertoire. What could happen is to silence them or turn them into regulatory or disease-protecting T cells.

Dr. Kalman: I don't believe that there is enough evidence to make this statement regarding humans. As described above in the case of bone marrow transplantation, this heroic strategy remains controversial today. In addition, T cells are essential elements of our immune system and would be generated again after the ablation and transplantation. It is uncertain how this new population of the host's lymphocytes might behave regarding autoimmunity.

37. *In the early 1990s there was research into monoclonal antibodies. What is the latest research on that?*

Dr. Olsson: Humanized monoclonal antibodies are now routinely used in the treatment of rheumatoid arthritis, directed against tumor necrosis factor alpha. They are tested in phase III trials, against an adhesion molecule in MS, with promising initial results. Thus, this tool is likely to be useful in the treatment of MS. Their role will depend on what target molecules in the pathogenesis will be defined.

Dr. Kaplin: Probably much of the unexpectedly poor response to some of the monoclonal antibody treatment in MS stems from the fact that these agents do not cross the blood-brain barrier and so cannot gain entry to the CNS where the damage takes place. Antegren, which works by blocking entry of immune cells into the CNS, may prove the most useful of this type of medication.

Dr. Weiner: A number of monoclonal antibodies are being tested in MS. The words *monoclonal antibody* are a general term and it depends on what the monoclonal antibody recognizes. I believe that different monoclonal antibodies will help patients with MS depending on what they are targeted against.

Dr. Kalman: Monoclonal antibodies are essential tools in modern medicine in several areas of diagnostics and therapy. Monoclonal antibodies are commonly used in diagnostics to better characterize abnormal cells or cellular/molecular components of tissue lesions. Monoclonal antibodies facilitate carrying out experiments testing how blocking or stimulation of certain pathways influence cell function. Recognition of the involvement of cell surface markers and adhesion molecules, cytokines, chemokines and matrix metalloproteinases in the process of MS prompted companies to develop monoclonal antibodies for the treatment of the disease by specifically targeting some of these molecules. A few among the most recently developed and tested therapeutical monoclonal antibodies include Antegren, CamPath, anti-CD4, anti-IL2, anti-IL2-receptor, rituximab, and others. While this is an exciting field, clinical trials are still necessary to establish the efficacy and long-term effects of these modalities.

Dr. Olek: Some trials were positive and some negative—they are still in the trial stage.

CURING MS

38. Over the past fifteen years, scientists and doctors have repeatedly predicted that MS would be cured "within five years." It's now 2004—is a cure in sight? Are you hopeful?

Dr. Olek: Yes, yes.

Dr. Moser: Not within five years.

Dr. Weiner: Depends on how one defines a cure. I think we already are helping control MS and I think better control over the disease indeed is in sight.

Dr. Kalman: The available drugs are becoming more and more potent. Several options can be considered now for each individual patient. However, I would not expect a cure until we fully understand the pathogenesis of the disease and try to target the cause. Even then, prevention and early treatment may be the most meaningful interventions. Nevertheless, we observe an overall acceleration in medical research and discoveries, which make all of us optimistic.

Dr. Kaplin: I am very hopeful for an eventual cure for all types of MS. In the next five to ten years I believe we can expect an increasingly useful armamentarium of medications to halt the progression in a majority of patients. Much like in the case of cancer, different forms of MS respond differently to treatment. Even with present suboptimal treatments we can get long-term remission in a minority of cases. Perhaps in five to ten years we will be able to put a majority of cases into long-term remission, but it may be the case that some difficult types of MS will elude effective management even over that time course. It is impossible to anticipate and keep major breakthroughs to a time schedule, however, and significant advances could prove right around the corner. Long-term hopes will undoubtedly depend on a commitment of resources to research in this area.

Dr. Olsson: It is very difficult to predict if there will be a complete cure or not. Today there are modifying treatments that are modestly effective against MS. This is important for several reasons. There are indeed treatments dampening MS. This has proven that it is possible to alter the natural course of the disease, and thereby encouraged attempts to find still better treatments. Pharmaceutical companies have seen that there is a profitable market for such drugs, encouraging them to further attempts. Now more drugs than ever are in the pipeline for MS. Many of them will fail, but it would be very surprising if some of them did not prove better then those existing today

I do not expect a sudden solution with a new treatment that will completely cure MS. Rather, I expect a stepwise improvement. This is what has been seen in other areas such as cancer. More and more forms of cancer are cured, but there are still challenges.

Dr. Frontera: Predictions are difficult to make but we have to remain hopeful!

39. How much money would you estimate it would take to put together a team or teams to devote full energy into finding a cure to MS?

Dr. Olek: $50 million to $100 million.

Dr. Weiner: This is a difficult question. Hundreds of millions of dollars are needed for the basic research that drives our understanding of MS. There are unique initiatives that I believe could be done.

Dr. Olsson: This is a very difficult question. Money is not enough, but it helps. Access to substantial funds will help to recruit the most talented and energetic researchers into this area. Furthermore, application to MS also depends on developments in immunology, genetics and neuroscience in general. Basic research on MS is relatively cheap as compared to clinical trials. This last matter is however best performed by the pharmaceutical industry, once proper targets have been defined in the more basic research. If I would be forced to give an estimate, I would guess that $500 million to $1 billion per year could be sufficient.

Dr. Kaplin: While resources are crucially important, it is the allocation of resources and attention to clinical topics that are also vital. There is a need for collaborative and interdisciplinary approaches. There is also the need to address all areas of vital relevance to the lives of MS patients. For example, there are precious few research dollars being spent on understanding and treating the biology of depression and cognitive impairment, even though the suffering and disability that these complications cause are devastating.

40. If you had that money, how would you spend it?

Dr. Olsson: Personally, I think that one of the most important topics is to find the genes, or the pathogenetic pathways regulated by them, allowing MS to evolve. As discussed, these are probably normal genes selected for during evolution, giving a side effect of disposing for MS. The genes would provide molecular targets that are more accessible for selective treatment. These genes may be difficult to find directly in humans with MS. However, with enough resources they can be positioned in mouse or rat models of MS. These genes, or genes along pathways controlled by these molecules, can then be studied on a large scale, using MS patients and control groups. Both the experimental work and subsequent work in humans are demanding of resources and time.

Dr. Olek: Clinical research with combination therapy.

Dr. Frontera: I would hire the best scientists in the field and would facilitate their collaboration by bringing them together and helping with their laboratory needs.

Dr. Kalman: I would like to integrate large-scale clinical, pathological, MRI, genetic and molecular studies, work in a team of experts, share resources and collaborate internationally.

Dr. Moser: Add to resources of existing teams; set priorities through peer-review mechanisms.

CONTROVERSIAL NONTRADITIONAL THERAPIES

41. Where do you stand on medical marijuana? Cooked or smoked or Marinol pills?

Dr. Olek: Legal in California; pills.

Dr. Olsson: Smoking gives cancer and is not advisable. If proper clinical trials with pills give data supporting pain relief in certain patients, I would prescribe it. As far as I know, such data are not yet available.

Dr. Weiner: If it is able to help people, I think it should be used.

Dr. Kalman: I think there are better standard alternatives.

Dr. Moser: I don't feel strongly. The importance of this discussion has been overblown. It needs careful evaluation.

42. *Where do you stand on herbal cures and other alternative medicine?*

Dr. Weiner: Some people gain benefit from these, however many of them are "quack" and some represent people trying to make money. Carefully used approaches may be helpful.

Dr. Kalman: Herbs and alternative medicine may have a complementary role in the management of MS, but cannot be the primary choice.

Dr. Olek: Okay as supplements to ABCR drugs (Avonex, Betaseron, Copaxone, Rebif).

Dr. Moser: There is no fundamental difference between alternative and other therapies.

43. *Would you recommend human growth hormones? Please explain why or why not.*

Dr. Olsson: At the moment, no. However, it is not excluded that growth hormone or other growth regulating factors in the future could be used in attempts to promote processes like remyelination. Once again, proper data is needed before giving therapy recommendations.

Dr. Olek: No—not rational for use.

Dr. Moser: Only if clinical trials indicate that it helps.

Dr. Weiner: The answer is no. I do not see how this could affect MS.

Dr. Kalman: I think we should primarily treat what we think is causally involved in the development of the disease. For symptomatic management I prefer to use well-established and harmless drugs. The biological effects of growth hormones and their involvement in neuroprotection or remyelination remain to be further investigated.

The Doctors' Credits

Dr. Walter R. Frontera

Walter R. Frontera, M.D., Ph.D., is an Associate Professor of Physical Medicine and Rehabilitation (PM&R) and Chairman of the Harvard Medical School Department of PM&R, and the Director of the Muscle Cell Physiology Laboratory at Spaulding Rehabilitation Hospital. He is a member of the Association of Academic Physiatrists, a Fellow in the Academy of Physical Medicine and Rehabilitation, a member of the American Physiological Society, and President of the Panamerican Confederation of Sports Medicine (COPAMEDE). He is a grant reviewer for the National Institutes of Health. In 2002 he was appointed the editor in chief of *The American Journal of Physical Medicine and Rehabilitation.*

His research interests include the effects of aging and exercise on skeletal muscle function and structure. Muscle weakness is a primary and secondary symptom of many diseases, including MS. Studies done by Dr. Frontera have been extended to include conditions such as inactivity and bed rest, and diseases affecting the central nervous system.

Dr. Bernadette Kalman

Assistant Professor of Neurology and Director of MS Research at St. Luke's–Roosevelt Hospital Center, Columbia University, Dr. Kalman received her M.D. degree summa cum laude and completed her board exam in clinical neurology with excellence in Hungary. Her postgraduate training involved a neuroimmunology fellowship at the Karolinska Institute, Stockholm, and at the Thomas Jefferson University, Philadelphia. She obtained her Ph.D. in immune genetics and neurogenetics.

Before moving to the SLRHC, she was a faculty member in the Department of Neurology of Thomas Jefferson University and Hahnemann University in Philadelphia. During the last few years she took two sabbaticals to study clinical features of neurogenetic diseases at the Institute of Neurology, Queen Square London, and genetic features of MS at the University of Oxford, Department of Clinical Neurology and the Wellcome Trust Center for Human Genetics in Oxford, England.

Her studies have been focused on clinical, immunological, molecular and genetic aspects of MS. She also studies genetic aspects of other neurological disorders. The main goal of her genetic studies is to identify susceptibility genes and to better understand the pathogenesis of the investigated diseases, primarily including MS. In addition, her group is currently developing a new project to identify markers of treatment response in MS, a new direction in the field of pharmacogenetics. She also participates in clinical studies and is involved in the development of an international MS database.

She has published close to fifty peer-reviewed articles and regularly gives lectures at scientific meetings around the world. She works in a broad international collaboration with clinician scientists in Central and Western Europe, Canada and the United States.

Dr. Adam Kaplin

Dr. Kaplin completed his undergraduate training at Yale University in 1988, where he graduated magna cum laude with a B.S. in Biology. He completed his M.D. and Ph.D. training at the Johns Hopkins School of Medicine in 1996, where he was a Medical Science Training Program awardee. Dr. Kaplin completed an internship in internal medicine at Johns Hopkins Bayview Medical Center, followed by residency training in psychiatry at Johns Hopkins Hospital. In his final year of residency training, he was selected to be Chief Resident of Psychiatry. Dr. Kaplin was invited to join the faculty as an Instructor in the Department of Psychiatry at Johns Hopkins School of Medicine immediately following his residency training, and was awarded one of the two Pfizer Postdoctoral Fellowship Grants in Biological Psychiatry offered in this country. In his second year on the faculty Dr. Kaplin was promoted to Assistant Professor of Psychiatry. Dr. Kaplin's research experience includes having been trained in the labs of two Nobel laureates and having completed his Ph.D. and postdoctoral training in the lab of Solomon Snyder, M.D., one of the preeminent leaders in the field of neuroscience and the founder of the Department of Neuroscience at Johns Hopkins. Additional awards that Dr. Kaplin has received include being selected as the NIH/NIMH Outstanding Resident of the year in 1998, and a Future Leader in Psychiatry Award by Emory University in 2002.

Dr. Kaplin has been an author on nine papers and six abstracts in scientific or medical journals. His research has focused on mechanisms of neuronal stimulation, communication and injury. He currently focuses on immune-mediated mechanisms of depression and cognitive impairment in multiple sclerosis and related autoimmune neurologic disorders, and the role of cytokines in these processes.

Since 1999 Dr. Kaplin has served as the Chief Psychiatric Consultant to the Multiple Sclerosis (MS) and Transverse Myelitis (TM) Centers at Johns Hopkins University School of Medicine. He is an integral member of the clinical and research endeavors of these centers, with an expertise in investigating the biological basis of depression and cognitive impairment in MS, and the care of patients afflicted with these complications. Dr. Kaplin is on the board of medical advisors to the Montel Williams MS Foundation and the International Transverse Myelitis Association.

Dr. Hugo W. Moser

Hugo W. Moser, M.D., is a research scientist and Director of the Neurogenetics Research Center at the Kennedy Krieger Institute. Dr. Moser is also University Professor of Neurology and Pediatrics at Johns Hopkins University. Dr. Moser serves on the editorial boards of *Journal of Neurosciences*, *Annals of Neurology*, *European Neurology* and other publications. Dr. Moser also has many professional memberships, consultant appointments, and publications. He has recently published papers in *Neurology*, *Brain and Development*, and the *American Journal of Human Genetics*.

Dr. Moser achieved international recognition for his research on genetic disorders that affect the nervous system function in children, particularly those that involve a part of the cell referred to as the peroxisome.

Dr. Michael J. Olek

Dr. Michael J. Olek recently joined UCI Medical Center's neurology department. Former director of clinical trials at the Multiple Sclerosis Center for Brigham and Women's/Massachusetts General Hospital, he now heads UCI Medical Center's Multiple Sclerosis Center. In this position, Olek plans to increase the research staff, perform clinical trials and enlarge the infusion unit.

A graduate of the Philadelphia College of Osteopathic Medicine, Olek completed a fellowship in clinical neuroimmunology at Harvard Medical School. For the past seven years, his research has focused on the pharmaceutical management of MS.

Olek sees such research as paving the way for future MS therapies and encourages community neurologists to refer their patients to his clinical studies. "Combination drug therapy is the direction we're going," he says. "Eventually, MS therapy will be like cancer therapy, with an emphasis on finding the right combination of drugs to effectively treat the disease, while reducing the side effects of cumulative toxicity."

Dr. Tomas Olsson

Dr. Tomas Olsson received his Ph.D. from the University of Linkoping and is currently director of the Department of Molecular Medicine at Karolinska Institute in Stockholm, Sweden. In addition, he is Professor of Molecular Medicine, and Senior Staff Physician in

Neurology. The coauthor of 236 original papers published or
accepted in internationally peer-reviewed journals, he is a member
of the Nobel assembly and a member of the editorial board of
Scandinavian Journal of Immunology and the *European Journal of
Neurology*.

Dr. Howard L. Weiner

Howard L. Weiner is the Robert L. Kroc Professor of Neurology at
Harvard Medical School and Director of the Multiple Sclerosis Center at the Brigham and Women's Hospital/Massachusetts General
Hospital. He is also Codirector of the Center for Neurologic Diseases at the Brigham and Women's Hospital. Dr. Weiner attended
Dartmouth College and received his M.D. from the University of
Colorado School of Medicine. He obtained his neurology training at
the Harvard Longwood neurology program. Following this, he pur-
sued his interest in immunology and virology as related to multiple
sclerosis. He has investigated basic and clinical aspects of autoimmunity in multiple sclerosis for the past twenty-five years. Dr. Weiner's
basic work has involved the study of viral interactions with the nervous system and the regulation of the immune system in the experimental model of multiple sclerosis and the use of mucosal tolerance
for the treatment of autoimmune diseases. Dr. Weiner has pioneered
the understanding of the mucosal immune system and how antigens
that are administered orally or nasally may be used to modulate
autoimmune and other inflammatory diseases. Based on his work,
oral vaccines have been tested not only in multiple sclerosis but also
in diabetes, arthritis and uveitis. The current trial of orally administered Copaxone to patients with multiple sclerosis is based on Dr.
Weiner's basic work on oral tolerance.

As part of his clinical investigations, Dr. Weiner has completed a
major study of MRI imaging in MS and has demonstrated linkage
of MRI abnormalities with different stages of MS. This has resulted
in a dynamic picture of the disease that had not previously been
observed.

Montel Williams has been a top player in the competitive daytime talk show arena since his debut in 1991. He is also a decorated former naval intelligence officer and a renowned motivational speaker, author, actor, and philanthropist. He is the creator of The Montel Williams MS Foundation.

Lawrence Grobel is the author of *Conversations with Capote; The Hustons; Conversations with Brando; Talking with Michener; Above the Line: Conversations About the Movies; Endangered Species: Writers Talk About Their Craft, Their Visions, Their Lives*; and *The Art of the Interview: Lessons from a Master of the Craft*. He is a contributing editor at *Playboy* and *Movieline's Hollywood Life* and has written for numerous national magazines and newspapers. *Playboy* called him "the interviewer's interviewer" and Joyce Carol Oates considers him "the Mozart of interviewers." He's served in the Peace Corps, received an NEA grant for fiction, and created the MFA in Professional Writing program for Antioch University. He currently teaches at UCLA.

The Montel Williams MS Foundation
331 West 57th Street, PMB #420
New York, NY 10019
www.montelms.org
212-830-0348

A portion of Montel's royalties from the sale of this
book are being donated to further MS research.